P

Handbook of
Surgical Technique

*A True Surgeon's Guide to Navigating
the Operating Room*

Handbook of Surgical Technique

A True Surgeon's Guide to Navigating the Operating Room

Christopher J. Hartman, MD
Assistant Professor of Urology
The Smith Institute for Urology
Hofstra-Northwell School of Medicine
Long Island, New York

Louis R. Kavoussi, MD, MBA
Waldbaum Gardiner Professor and Chairman
The Smith Institute for Urology
Hofstra-Northwell School of Medicine
Long Island, New York

ELSEVIER

ELSEVIER

1600 John F. Kennedy Blvd.
Ste 1800
Philadelphia, PA 19103-2899

HANDBOOK OF SURGICAL TECHNIQUES   ISBN: 978-0-323-46201-3

Notices

Knowledge and best practice in this field are constantly changing. As new research and experience broaden our understanding, changes in research methods, professional practices, or medical treatment may become necessary.

Practitioners and researchers must always rely on their own experience and knowledge in evaluating and using any information, methods, compounds, or experiments described herein. In using such information or methods they should be mindful of their own safety and the safety of others, including parties for whom they have a professional responsibility.

With respect to any drug or pharmaceutical products identified, readers are advised to check the most current information provided (i) on procedures featured or (ii) by the manufacturer of each product to be administered, to verify the recommended dose or formula, the method and duration of administration, and contraindications. It is the responsibility of practitioners, relying on their own experience and knowledge of their patients, to make diagnoses, to determine dosages and the best treatment for each individual patient, and to take all appropriate safety precautions.

To the fullest extent of the law, neither the Publisher nor the authors, contributors, or editors, assume any liability for any injury and/or damage to persons or property as a matter of products liability, negligence or otherwise, or from any use or operation of any methods, products, instructions, or ideas contained in the material herein.

Library of Congress Cataloging-in-Publication Data

Names: Hartman, Christopher J., author. | Kavoussi, Louis R., author.
Title: Handbook of surgical technique : a true surgeon's guide to navigating the operating room / Christopher J. Hartman, Louis R. Kavoussi.
Description: Philadelphia, PA : Elsevier, [2018] | Includes bibliographical
    references and index.
Identifiers: LCCN 2017038058| ISBN 9780323462013 (pbk. : alk. paper) | ISBN 9780826169334 (e-book)
Subjects: | MESH: Surgical Procedures, Operative--methods | Operating Rooms
Classification: LCC RD32.3 | NLM WO 500 | DDC 617.9/17--dc23 LC record available at https://lccn.loc.gov/2017038058

Executive Content Strategist: James T. Merritt
Content Development Specialist: Meghan Andress
Publishing Services Manager: Catherine Jackson
Project Manager: Tara Delaney
Design Direction: Bridget Hoette

Printed in China

Last digit is the print number: 9   8   7   6   5   4   3   2   1

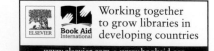

To my wife, Kerri,
without whose unfaltering support, love, and dedication
this would not have been possible.

CJH

This is dedicated to my surgical mentors
Bill Catalona, Ralph Clayman,
Jerry Andriole, and Herb Lepor,
whose voices echo in every incision made
and stitch thrown.

LRK

PREFACE

In every technical field, it is important to understand and master fundamentals. The surgical arts are no exception to this requirement. Those wishing to be involved in the care of patients need to be grounded in the culture, resources, and processes of the operating room. Thus far, there have been a limited number of resources available to students that provide a comprehensive overview of these fundamentals. Most gain familiarity through a "trial by fire" approach, where there is great variability in experiences, and holes in an individual's basic education can persist for years.

This text was born out of a need to help students gain a cardinal knowledge of the workings of the operating room and smoothly integrate into the surgical team. This handbook covers the basic protocol and culture of the operating room to help students understand the purpose of roles within the operating room as well as the behaviors needed to excel. Equipment and tools are reviewed, and the rationale for use of each is described. Basic techniques in surgery are explained, and tips are provided to allow a new individual in the operating room to assist in a meaningful way.

This text offers a concise yet comprehensive review of the operating room, its components, and how to excel in surgery. We encourage you to review the online videos that complement this book, which demonstrate and explain various surgical techniques in more depth. We hope you enjoy the art of surgery, and we will see you in the operating room!

Christopher J. Hartman, MD
Louis R. Kavoussi, MD, MBA

ACKNOWLEDGMENTS

We wish to acknowledge the countless OR nurses, physicians assistants, and surgical residents at Long Island Jewish Medical Center and North Shore University Hospital who aided in gathering supplies, served as the subjects for a number of photographs, and provided inspiration for writing this book. We are especially indebted to Saramma Sam, Wayland Wu, and Vinaya Vasudevan, who were integral in this process. We also wish to thank Riccardo Galli and David Leavitt, without whose skill and dedication to the videography portion of this text, this work would not have been possible.

Finally, we have to thank the remarkable editorial staff at Elsevier. James Merritt understood the importance of this text and helped with organizing and advocating for its production. Meghan Andress was essential in operationalizing the project as well as keeping us on track. We also need to give tremendous thanks to a master "cat herder" Tara Delaney, our project manager, who brought this opus home. We are grateful to Elsevier for not only believing in the need for this textbook, but for also helping to create it.

Christopher J. Hartman, MD
Louis R. Kavoussi, MD, MBA

CONTENTS

VIDEO CONTENTS

INTRODUCTION: THE SURGICAL CULTURE

The operating room (OR) is an entirely unique experience. It requires a strict adherence to sterility, attention to detail, and precision to optimize outcomes. Minor mistakes or lapses in judgment can result in detrimental or even fatal outcomes. For this reason, each member of the OR team has a vital role in ensuring patient safety and security. From the nursing staff who operationalize the environment to the anesthesiologist entrusted to securing the airway, keeping the patient asleep during the procedure, and perioperative pain control, to the medical student tasked with retraction, suctioning, or holding the camera during laparoscopic procedures, to the cleaning staff assigned to ensuring a clean and sterile environment for subsequent patients after a procedure has been completed, all individuals play an integral role in promoting patient safety and timely delivery of high-quality medical care. It is for these reasons that special rules and regulations apply within the OR.

The OR can be a daunting place for the uninitiated. From a simple incision and drainage of an abscess to the more complex Whipple procedure, each case presents its own unique set of challenges. As such, surgery—including not only operative skill but also knowledge of a myriad of diseases and their associated pathology, anatomy, and physiology—can be an overwhelming experience for all. From a medical student's very first foray into the OR to a surgeon's last case as an attending physician, patients entrust their lives and well-being to the surgeon's knowledge and skill. Fortunately, the evolution of the field of medicine to include a culture of transparency and team-based approaches has made surgery safer for patients and has eased students' introduction to the operating theater.

A notable example of the team at work is in the preparation of the patient on the operating table. After induction of anesthesia, meticulous care is taken by all members of the team to take a human in his most vulnerable state and maintain that person's dignity in the safest manner. Positioning involves checks and balances to optimize the operative field for the surgeon and secure vascular access and physiologic monitoring for the anesthesiologist, all while mitigating pressure or stretch injuries to the patient. Additionally, several steps are taken to minimize the risks of infectious complications during surgery by creating a sterile field.

Skin or epithelial surface disinfection, meticulous handwashing, sterile processing and assessing the cleanliness of equipment, and sterile draping of the patient are components that require a group effort. Although it is the responsibility of the surgeon and other individuals who are scrubbed for a procedure to maintain a local sterile field, all members of the surgical team have a duty to not only adhere to strict sterile principles but also to immediately report when a break in sterility occurs.

The delivery of medical care requires a collaborative and multifaceted approach; however, in the OR, a single attending surgeon typically serves as the quarterback who directs others during the surgery. Not only does the surgeon dictate the operative course, but he also sets the tone for all. Is it a particularly stressful case, such as a trauma where time is of the essence and the surgeon's body language demands quick responses from the surgical assistant, scrub technician, and circulator? Is it a novel or rare case in which, along with treating the patient, educating residents, medical students, and other trainees is vital to ensure future delivery of medical care? Multiple factors, including patient age, body habitus, comorbidities, technical difficulty of the case, and the severity of the disease collaborate to impact a surgeon's tone in the OR. It is therefore also the role of the surgeon to lead by example, and how he or she treats the other members of the surgical team can either positively or negatively affect patient care. A relaxed, respectful, yet confident surgeon can allow others in the OR to concentrate on their role and responsibilities throughout a surgery, whereas one who is more demanding, unfriendly, or even derogatory toward staff members can negatively affect patient care by leaving others thinking more about being chastised for doing something wrong than aiding throughout the surgery.

Surgeons, as opposed to other physicians and medical professionals, are typically regarded as being very goal driven and focused. Fig. 1 presents 12 different personality traits and how they differ between internists and surgeons, as assessed by nurses and through physician self-assessment. There were no statistically

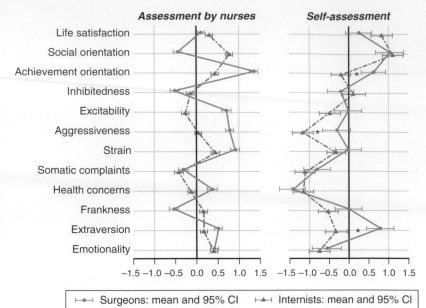

Fig. 1 Personality traits of surgeons compared to internists, as assessed by nurses and physician self-report. Reproduced with permission from Warschkow R, Steffen T, Spillmann M, Kolb W, Lange J, Tarantino I. A comparative cross-sectional study of personality traits in internists and surgeons. *Surgery.* 2010;148(5):901–907.

significant differences in personality as assessed by nurses; however, via self-assessment, surgeons reported being more achievement oriented and extraverted than internists, whereas internists reported being less aggressive than surgeons.[1] These personality differences often develop prior to medical training, and medical students interested in surgery frequently report being drawn to the field due to these characteristics, which they observe in attending surgeons and surgical residents.[2,3]

The aim of this handbook is to provide a quick, concise review of surgical principles, techniques, instruments, and supplies commonly encountered in the OR. When is a cutting needle preferred over a noncutting needle? In what circumstances are nonabsorbable sutures necessary as opposed to absorbable sutures?

Where should a toothed forceps be used instead of a blunt forceps? What is the role of all other nonscrubbed individuals in the OR? A discussion of the complex culture of the OR follows, addressing these and a multitude of other questions.

REFERENCES

1. Warschkow R, Steffen T, Spillmann M, Kolb W, Lange J, Tarantino I. A comparative cross-sectional study of personality traits in internists and surgeons. *Surgery.* 2010;148(5):901–907.
2. O'Herrin JK, Lewis BJ, Rikkers LF, Chen H. Why do students choose careers in surgery? *Journal of Surgical Research.* 2004;119(2):124–129.
3. Scott IM, Matejcek AN, Gowans MC, Wright BJ, Brenneis FR. Choosing a career in surgery: factors that influence Canadian medical students' interest in pursuing a surgical career. *Canadian Journal of Surgery.* 2008;51(5):371–377.

CHAPTER 1

PREOPERATIVE PREPARATION OF THE PATIENT

Attention to preoperative preparation is pivotal in mitigating surgical risk. As medical science has improved survival, more patients are now candidates for surgical cure. Comorbidities, such as hypertension, cardiac disease, and diabetes mellitus, are becoming increasingly more prevalent in patients, and therefore optimization of health lowers possible risk prior to a surgical procedure. The goal of presurgical testing and medical evaluation is to both optimize existing comorbidities and uncover previously undiagnosed illness that may adversely affect perioperative outcomes.[1] The preoperative preparation must accordingly be tailored to each individual patient based on several factors including age, medical comorbidities, anesthetic risk, and the proposed surgical procedure. For instance, a healthy 35-year-old patient undergoing excision of a skin lesion under anesthesia requires less preoperative preparation than a 70-year-old patient with diverticulitis, congestive heart failure, and chronic kidney disease set to undergo a colon resection. Preoperative preparation encompasses the various laboratory tests, imaging studies, and medical clearances a patient must undergo prior to surgery.

There has been significant work in finding a balance between overtesting and trivializing risk. The American Society of Anesthesiologists (ASA) has developed the ASA physical status (ASA PS) classification system, a validated system aimed at assigning anesthetic risk to patients undergoing surgical procedures (Table 1.1). First introduced in 1941, it has since undergone multiple revisions and can be applied to patients undergoing both elective and emergent procedures.[2] Although an adverse outcome can occur in any patient undergoing anesthesia, the risk for a major event generally increases as ASA PS class increases. It is important to discuss these and operation-specific risks with patients prior to any procedure.

PREOPERATIVE EVALUATION

In general, preoperative preparation should begin with a thorough evaluation by the surgeon to assess the need for surgical intervention. For example, whereas a nontoxic patient with a small kidney stone may be able to pass the stone without intervention, a patient with a large obstructing ureteral calculus with signs and symptoms of sepsis likely needs a procedure to decompress the urinary system. This determination is made by the surgeon.

Determining the type of surgery to be performed is also tasked to the surgeon. A vascular surgeon may suggest performing an endovascular abdominal aortic aneurysm (AAA) repair in a patient with numerous medical comorbidities compared to an open AAA repair in a younger, healthier patient. These decisions are made together with the patient and may require the expertise of other practitioners, such as primary medical providers who help assess the medical risk of surgery.

After evaluating a patient for surgery, the remainder of the preoperative clearance evaluation should be determined by patient comorbidities. In general, patients with lung disease such as interstitial or restrictive lung diseases may need pulmonary clearance, whereas patients with significant cardiac comorbidities such as coronary artery disease (CAD) or congestive heart failure will require evaluation by a cardiologist. Although different centers have different requirements for when a patient needs medical clearance, it is generally accepted that healthy, low-risk patients undergoing low- to moderate-risk surgical procedures do not need a formal preoperative clearance by a medical doctor. Consideration for preoperative clearance in older individuals, however, should be based on the morbidity of the surgery to be performed. Patients with extensive medical comorbidities should always be cleared medically prior to surgery.

Although advanced age in itself should not be used to assess surgical risk, numerous studies have examined the effect of advanced age on surgical outcomes. In general, a slight increase in risk has been demonstrated with advancing age,[3,4] and one study found a positive linear relationship between mortality and increasing age for most surgical procedures.[5] As older individuals are more likely to have more significant medical comorbidities,

Table 1.1 American Society of Anesthesiologists Physical Status Classification System

ASA PS Classification*	Definition	Examples (Including but Not Limited To)
ASA I	A normal healthy patient	Healthy, nonsmoking, no or minimal alcohol use.
ASA II	A patient with mild systemic disease	Mild diseases only without substantive functional limitations. Examples include (but are not limited to) current smoker, social alcohol drinker, pregnancy, obesity (30 < BMI <40), well-controlled DM/HTN, mild lung disease.
ASA III	A patient with severe systemic disease	Substantive functional limitations; one or more moderate to severe diseases. Examples include (but are not limited to) poorly controlled DM or HTN, COPD, morbid obesity (BMI ≥40), active hepatitis, alcohol dependence or abuse, implanted pacemaker, moderate reduction of ejection fraction, ESRD undergoing regularly scheduled dialysis, premature infant PCA <60 weeks, history (>3 months) of MI, CVA, TIA, or CAD/stents.
ASA IV	A patient with severe systemic disease that is a constant threat to life	Examples include (but are not limited to) recent (<3 months) MI, CVA, TIA, or CAD/stents, ongoing cardiac ischemia or severe valve dysfunction, severe reduction of ejection fraction, sepsis, DIC, ARD, or ESRD not undergoing regularly scheduled dialysis.
ASA V	A moribund patient who is not expected to survive without the operation	Examples include (but are not limited to) ruptured abdominal/thoracic aneurysm, massive trauma, intracranial bleed with mass effect, ischemic bowel in the face of significant cardiac pathology or multiple organ/system dysfunction.
ASA VI	A declared brain-dead patient whose organs are being removed for donor purposes	

*The addition of "E" denotes emergency surgery (an emergency is defined as existing when delay in treatment of the patient would lead to a significant increase in the threat to life or body part).
ASA PS, American Society of Anesthesiologists physical status; ASA, American Society of Anesthesiologists; BMI, body mass index; DM, diabetes mellitus; HTN, hypertension; COPD, chronic obstructive pulmonary disease; ESRD, end-stage renal disease; PCA, patient-controlled analgesia; MI, myocardial infarction; CVA, cerebrovascular accident; TIA, transient ischemic attack; CAD, coronary artery disease; DIC, disseminated intravascular coagulation; ARD, advanced renal disease.
Reproduced with permission from http://www.asahq.org/resources/clinical-information/asa-physical-status-classification-system

both age and overall health status should be used in assessing surgical risk.

Preoperative Cardiovascular Evaluation

Of particular importance when evaluating a patient for surgery is the preoperative cardiovascular assessment. It has been estimated that nearly 30% of patients undergoing surgical procedures have some degree of CAD or other cardiac comorbidity. Therefore, in addition to uncovering previously unknown cardiac disease, it is essential to determine the severity and relative stability of preexisting cardiac disease. The American College of Cardiology (ACC) and American Heart Association (AHA) have developed guidelines to be used for perioperative cardiac evaluation prior to surgery.[6] Clinical risk for perioperative adverse cardiac outcomes is generally based on a patient's functional capacity, the type of surgery to be performed, and specific clinical markers.[7]

Functional capacity, typically evaluated in metabolic equivalents (METs), is a marker of a patient's ability to meet metabolic demands for certain activities. Table 1.2 presents the Duke Activity Status Index, which quantifies a number of common activities with their associated METs.[8] It is generally accepted that a patient who can comfortably perform activities that require >4 METs, such as light housework, climbing a flight of stairs, or walking four blocks on level ground, has a lower cardiac risk for perioperative adverse outcomes.[9,10] In addition, the ACC/AHA has published practice guidelines and clinical predictors of increased perioperative cardiovascular risk, which are presented in Box 1.1.

Table 1.2 Duke Activity Status Index

Item	Activity	Weight
1	Can you take care of yourself (eating, dressing, bathing, or using the toilet)?	2.75
2	Can you walk indoors, such as around your house?	1.75
3	Can you walk a block or two on level ground?	2.75
4	Can you climb a flight of stairs or walk up a hill?	5.50
5	Can you run a short distance?	8.00
6	Can you do light work around the house like dusting or washing dishes?	2.70
7	Can you do moderate work around the house like vacuuming, sweeping floors, or carrying in groceries?	3.50
8	Can you do heavy work around the house like scrubbing floors, or lifting and moving heavy furniture?	8.00
9	Can you do yard work like raking leaves, weeding, or pushing a power mower?	4.50
10	Can you have sexual relations?	5.25
11	Can you participate in moderate recreational activities like golf, bowling, dancing, doubles tennis, or throwing a baseball or football?	6.00
12	Can you participate in strenuous sports like swimming, singles tennis, football, basketball, or skiing?	7.50

Modified from Hlatky MA, Boineau RE, Higginbotham MB, et al. A brief self-administered questionnaire to determine functional capacity (the Duke Activity Status Index). American Journal of Cardiology. 1989;64(10):651-654.

The type of surgery to be performed also has a substantial impact on a patient's perioperative cardiovascular risk. Vascular surgeries and complicated

---

Box 1.1 Clinical Predictors of Increased Perioperative Cardiovascular Risk

Major

Unstable coronary syndromes
- Acute or recent myocardial infarction with evidence of important ischemic risk by clinical symptoms or noninvasive study
- Unstable or severe angina (Canadian class III or IV)

Decompensated heart failure

Significant arrhythmias
- High-grade atrioventricular block
- Symptomatic ventricular arrhythmias in the presence of underlying heart disease
- Supraventricular arrhythmias with uncontrolled ventricular rate

Severe valvular disease

Intermediate

Mild angina pectoris (Canadian class I or II)

Previous myocardial infarction by history or pathological Q waves

Compensated or prior heart failure

Diabetes mellitus (particularly insulin dependent)

Renal insufficiency

Minor

Advanced age

Abnormal EKG (left ventricular hypertrophy, left bundle-branch block, ST-T abnormalities)

Rhythm other than sinus (e.g., atrial fibrillation)

Low functional capacity (e.g., inability to climb one flight of stairs with a bag of groceries)

History of stroke

Uncontrolled systemic hypertension

Reproduced with permission from Eagle KA, Berger PB, Calkins H, et al. ACC/AHA guideline update for perioperative cardiovascular evaluation for noncardiac surgery—executive summary. A report of the American College of Cardiology/American Heart Association Task Force on Practice Guidelines (Committee to Update the 1996 Guidelines on Perioperative Cardiovascular Evaluation for Noncardiac Surgery). *Circulation.* 2002;105(10):1257-1267.

Box 1.2 Cardiac Risk Stratification for Noncardiac Surgical Procedures

High (reported cardiac risk often >5%)
- Emergent major operations, particularly in the elderly
- Aortic and other major vascular surgery
- Peripheral vascular surgery
- Anticipated prolonged surgical procedures associated with large fluid shifts and/or blood loss

Intermediate (reported cardiac risk generally <5%)
- Carotid endarterectomy
- Head and neck surgery
- Intraperitoneal and intrathoracic surgery
- Orthopedic surgery
- Prostate surgery

Low (reported cardiac risk generally <1%)
- Endoscopic procedures
- Superficial procedure
- Cataract surgery
- Breast surgery

Reproduced with permission from Eagle KA, Berger PB, Calkins H, et al. ACC/AHA guideline update for perioperative cardiovascular evaluation for noncardiac surgery—executive summary. A report of the American College of Cardiology/American Heart Association Task Force on Practice Guidelines (Committee to Update the 1996 Guidelines on Perioperative Cardiovascular Evaluation for Noncardiac Surgery). *Circulation.* 2002;105(10):1257-1267.

---

procedures with the potential for large blood loss and longer operative time carry a greater cardiovascular risk than minor procedures. The ACC/AHA practice guidelines also stratify surgery type by risk, which is presented in Box 1.2.

Cardiac evaluation prior to surgery begins with cardiac auscultation, which evaluates for murmurs, arrhythmias, and extra heart sounds. Auscultation should be performed during any cardiac workup prior to surgery. Additional testing should be performed at the discretion of the evaluating cardiologist and may include electrocardiography (EKG), echocardiography, and stress testing (see the Special Testing section). ACC/AHA practice guidelines direct clinicians on which tests to perform and are updated regularly to reflect best practice guidelines.[6]

Preoperative Pulmonary Evaluation

Although rare, postoperative pulmonary complications can be devastating, life threatening, and extremely costly. Significant comorbid pulmonary diseases, such as obstructive sleep apnea (OSA), chronic obstructive pulmonary disease (COPD), asthma, and pulmonary hypertension are commonly encountered in surgical patients. It is therefore extremely important to optimize a patient's pulmonary status to avert preventable complications. Risk factors for patient-related pulmonary complications after surgery include advanced age,[11] COPD,[12] smoking,[13] obesity,[14] and heart failure,[15] among others. Numerous procedure-related factors can also have an impact on pulmonary complications postoperatively. Longer procedures typically have a greater risk for pulmonary compromise, as well as surgeries involving the chest or upper abdomen.

In evaluating a patient who is to undergo surgery, the most important element in the preoperative pulmonary assessment is a thorough history and physical examination.[16] Patients with no prior pulmonary history typically do not need preoperative risk stratification or evaluation by a pulmonologist except for patients undergoing planned thoracic procedures. The ARISCAT risk index (Table 1.3) offers a convenient way of estimating a patient's postoperative pulmonary risk after surgery.[17] In general, patients deemed to be at low risk for postoperative pulmonary complications do not need additional pulmonary testing, whereas patients deemed to be at high risk should be evaluated by a pulmonologist. Pulmonary function tests (PFTs) have utility in patients with preexisting pulmonary disease to assess the severity of impairment prior to undergoing a surgical procedure. PFTs should also be performed in patients undergoing thoracic procedures, especially in cases in which lung volume reduction is planned.

Table 1.3 ARISCAT Risk Index: Independent Predictors of Postoperative Pulmonary Complications

Factor	Adjusted Odds Ratio (95% CI)	Risk Score
Age (years)		
≤50	1	
51-80	1.4 (0.6-3.3)	3
>80	5.1 (1.9-13.3)	16
Preoperative O$_2$ saturation		
≥96%	1	
91-95%	2.2 (1.2-4.2)	8
≤90%	10.7 (4.1-28.1)	24
Respiratory infection in the past month	5.5 (2.6-11.5)	17
Preoperative anemia, hemoglobin ≤10 g/dL	3 (1.4-6.5)	11
Surgical incision		
Upper abdominal	4.4 (2.3-8.5)	15
Intrathoracic	11.4 (1.9-26.0)	24
Duration of surgery		
≤2 hours	1	
2-3 hours	4.9 (2.4-10.1)	16
>3 hours	9.7 (2.4-19.9)	23
Emergency surgery	2.2 (1.0-4.5)	8

Risk Class (Validation Sample)	Number of Points in Risk Score	Pulmonary Complication Rate
Low	<26 points	1.6%
Intermediate	26-44 points	13.3%
High	≥45 points	42.1%

Modified from Canet J, Gallart L, Gomar C, et al. Prediction of postoperative pulmonary complications in a population-based surgical cohort. Anesthesiology. 2010;113(6):1338-1350.

LABORATORY DATA

Although there is not a standard approach to preoperative laboratory testing, each center typically mandates some degree of preoperative testing in adults prior to surgery. In general, it is rare to find an abnormality that will affect surgery itself; however, in many instances such testing serves as a baseline in the event of an unexpected complication or outcome. Preoperative laboratory testing usually includes a complete blood count (CBC), basic metabolic panel (BMP), and coagulation studies (prothrombin time/international normalized ratio [PT/INR], partial thromboplastin time [PTT]). Other laboratory tests are typically ordered as indicated based on surgery and patient-related factors.[18] In female patients of reproductive age, urine or blood for human chorionic growth hormone (HCG) testing is obtained, as significant pregnancy complications can occur to a developing fetus if pregnancy is not recognized. Thus, HCG testing should be performed in women of reproductive age on the day of any surgical procedure that requires anesthesia.

In the absence of any identifiable clinical risk factors for anesthesia, some groups have advocated for limited or no laboratory testing prior to surgery. Recent practice guidelines from the ASA, for example, specifically recommend against laboratory testing in patients without identifiable indications to do so.[19]

A CBC has utility in preoperative testing for several reasons. Patients with a history of anemia, older patients, or those undergoing surgeries with the potential for significant blood loss could benefit from diagnosing underlying anemia. Preoperative anemia has been found to predict postoperative mortality, even in the absence of significant intraoperative blood loss.[20] Additionally, in patients having a planned spinal or epidural anesthesia, it is important to evaluate for thrombocytopenia to minimize the potential for intrathecal bleeding.

Preoperative BMP testing has utility in detecting underlying renal disease or assessing stability of preexisting renal impairment via creatinine measurements, detecting electrolyte abnormalities, and uncovering unrecognized diabetes. Renal impairment has been correlated with postoperative cardiac and pulmonary complications, as well as increased postoperative mortality.[15,21,22]

Although preoperative electrolyte abnormalities are exceedingly rare, preoperative hypernatremia has been associated with significant postoperative morbidity and mortality.[23] Underlying hypernatremia can often be discerned by a thorough history, such as inquiring about diuretic or angiotensin-converting enzyme inhibitor use. Thus, routine electrolyte evaluation is not recommended for most patients but is usually included in a BMP.

Hyper- and hypokalemia also can have devastating consequences on surgical outcomes. Both can lead to serious cardiac arrhythmias that are exacerbated by anesthesia. Both are exceedingly rare, however, outside of patients who are extremely malnourished or have renal impairment. Isolated potassium testing is therefore not recommended in healthy individuals.

Diabetes can have a significant impact on wound healing and is also associated with cardiac complications and postoperative mortality. Blood glucose testing, however, is not a reliable measure of diabetes control. In patients with diabetes, and particularly in patients for whom the concern of poor diabetes control exists, a hemoglobin A1c (HbA1c) level should be obtained. Elevated blood glucose levels may prompt an evaluation for unrecognized diabetes but should not be routinely obtained as part of the preoperative workup in most patients.

Coagulation studies, including PT/INR and PTT, should not routinely be obtained in healthy patients prior to surgery. If no prior family history of a bleeding disorder exists, and the history and physical exam do not suggest a bleeding disorder, the utility of coagulation studies is very limited. In the case of a patient on an anticoagulant, such as warfarin or enoxaparin,

Table 1.4   Summary of Typical Laboratory Studies Obtained Prior to Surgery

Test	Abbreviation	Components	Use in Presurgical Testing
Complete blood count	CBC	White blood cell count (WBC)	Evaluation for infection
		Hemoglobin	Evaluation for anemia
		Hematocrit	Evaluation for anemia
		Platelet count	Evaluation for impaired blood clotting ability
Basic metabolic panel	BMP/Chem 7	Sodium (Na)	Evaluation for hyper- or hyponatremia
		Potassium (K)	Evaluation for hyper- or hypokalemia
		Chloride (Cl)	
		Bicarbonate (HCO_3^-)	Evaluation for acidosis/alkalosis
		Blood urea nitrogen (BUN)	Evaluation for renal impairment
		Creatinine (Cr)	Evaluation for renal impairment
		Glucose (G)	
Prothrombin time/international normalized ratio	PT/INR		Evaluation for impaired blood clotting
Partial thromboplastin time	PTT		Evaluation for impaired blood clotting
Human chorionic growth hormone	HCG		Pregnancy testing
Urine culture	UCx		Evaluation for urinary tract infection

coagulation studies are indicated. Additionally, in patients who are planned to undergo complex, prolonged procedures with the potential for high blood loss, baseline coagulation studies may be obtained.

In general, urine studies such as a urinalysis and urine culture should not be obtained prior to most surgical procedures. In patients with symptoms of a urinary tract infection, however, a urinalysis and urine culture may be indicated. Additionally, for procedures with planned entry into the genitourinary tract, a urinalysis and urine culture should be obtained. Table 1.4 summarizes the typical components of preoperative laboratory evaluation.

SPECIAL TESTING

Numerous additional tests are available to aid in evaluation of risk prior to surgery. Common tests include the EKG, chest x-ray (CXR), echocardiogram, cardiac stress testing, and PFTs. Of these, an EKG and CXR are most commonly obtained prior to surgery, with some centers still requiring them to be performed, despite recommendations against their use for minor surgical procedures in otherwise healthy individuals.[6] One study estimated that the rates of EKG testing prior to low-risk procedures are highly variable among different institutions, with some centers obtaining an EKG in as few as 3.4% of patients and others obtaining it in as many as 88.8% of patients.[24]

Much of the debate over whether to obtain an EKG prior to surgery stems from the limited information it offers in patients without a prior cardiac history. Certain studies have demonstrated routine EKG testing to be of no predictive value,[25] whereas others argue that an EKG is the best diagnostic test to predict adverse cardiac events postoperatively.[26] Most physicians would

agree that an EKG should be obtained prior to surgery in patients with a significant cardiac history to assess stability and to have a baseline study in the event of postoperative problems. In patients without preexisting cardiac disease, however, and especially in patients younger than 40 years, EKG testing is unlikely to reveal any abnormalities and in most cases is unnecessary and only adds extra cost to the preoperative workup.

The decision as to whether to obtain a CXR has equally been debated. In patients with a history of COPD, asthma, OSA, or other respiratory disease, a CXR should be obtained, but without preexisting cardiopulmonary disease, it is controversial as to whether a CXR should be obtained. In patients undergoing prolonged surgical procedures that require intubation, a preoperative CXR allows for later comparison should a postoperative cardiopulmonary complication arise. Preoperative screening CXRs, however, have not been correlated with morbidity and mortality, and therefore should not be routinely obtained prior to most surgical procedures.[27]

An echocardiogram can be useful in patients undergoing planned cardiac procedures but is not routinely obtained in healthy patients. Patients with cardiac comorbidities, however, such as congestive heart failure or valvular heart disease, may benefit from preoperative echocardiography to assess cardiac function and stability of preexisting disease. In patients with overall poor health status and concern for significant anesthetic risks, preoperative cardiac stress testing may help to define which patients are fit to undergo surgery in comparison to those who are not. In general, a cardiologist or pulmonologist should evaluate patients with significant cardiac and pulmonary comorbidities prior to surgery, and the decision to order specific tests should be at the discretion of those providers.

PATIENT PREPARATION

The specific type of preparation that a patient should undergo prior to surgery typically depends on the type of surgery to be performed. This includes bowel preparation, antibiotic use, and cessation of certain medications such as anticoagulants, diabetes medications, and antihypertensives. Additionally, all patients undergoing elective surgeries should fast prior to the procedure. In patients undergoing emergency procedures, the benefits of fasting must be weighed against the risk of prolonging the interval to surgery. Thus, in some patients who present with surgical emergencies, requirements for fasting are usurped by the urgency of the procedure.

The ASA recommends different lengths of fasting for different types of ingested foods and liquid. These recommendations are summarized in Table 1.5 and are based on gastric emptying time. In general, clear liquids comprise liquids such as water, fruit juices without pulp, sports drinks, coffee, clear tea, and carbonated beverages, and the minimum period of fasting should be at least 2 hours prior to undergoing surgery. For infants who are breast-feeding, no breast milk should be ingested for at least 4 hours prior to surgery. Infant formula, however, should be restricted for at least 6 hours prior to surgery due to its longer gastric emptying time. Nonhuman milk should be restricted in children and adults for a minimum of at least 6 hours prior to surgery. A light meal, such as that which consists of toast and clear liquids, should not be eaten within at least 6 hours of a surgical procedure. Fatty foods require a longer gastric transit time and therefore should not be ingested for at least 8 hours prior to surgery. These are general recommendations for fasting; however, the ASA cautions that not only the type but also the quantity of food ingested should be considered when determining an appropriate fasting interval.[28]

Restricting anticoagulant and antiplatelet agents prior to surgery should be based on several procedure- and patient-related factors. For procedures in which the estimated blood loss is relatively minimal, patients with a high risk of thromboembolic events or recently placed cardiac stents should typically continue their medications throughout the perioperative period. For procedures with a high risk of blood loss, antiplatelet agents such as aspirin or clopidogrel may need to be stopped prior to the procedure. The length of discontinuation will depend on the half-life of the medication. As data is becoming available, more surgeries are being performed on limited antiplatelet agents, such as aspirin. A thorough evaluation of the risk and benefits of discontinuing aspirin and clopidogrel should be undertaken when deciding whether to hold or continue them in the perioperative period.

Table 1.5	Summary of American Society of Anesthesiologists Recommendations for Fasting Prior to Anesthesia	
Ingested Material	**Minimum Fasting Period**
Clear liquids	2 hours
Breast milk	4 hours
Infant formula	6 hours
Nonhuman milk	6 hours
Light meal	6 hours

Modified from Apfelbaum J, Caplan R, Connis R, Epstein B, Nickinovich D, Warner M. Practice guidelines for preoperative fasting and the use of pharmacologic agents to reduce the risk of pulmonary aspiration: application to healthy patients undergoing elective procedures. An updated report by the American Society of Anesthesiologists Committee on Standards and Practice Parameters. Anesthesiology. 2011;114(3):495-511.

In general, warfarin should be stopped at an appropriate interval prior to surgery, and PT/INR levels should be checked immediately prior to surgery to minimize bleeding risk. In patients with a high risk of thromboembolic events, the risk of bleeding must be carefully weighed against the risk of stroke or other potentially devastating complication. In certain patients for whom the risk of perioperative bleeding and a thromboembolic event is high, such as those patients with previous or current deep venous thrombosis or a pulmonary embolism, stopping anticoagulation and the placement of a permanent or retrievable inferior vena cava filter should be considered.

Mechanical bowel preparation (MBP) may be necessary in certain types of surgery, such as those that require entry into the gastrointestinal tract. The use of MBP for routine intraabdominal procedures without planned entry into the gastrointestinal tract may also be considered based on the complexity of the case as well as surgeon preference. Risks of MBP include dehydration and falls in patients who are elderly, as well as patient discomfort, and therefore should be used with caution. MBP may be achieved via several different methods. Polyethylene glycol solutions, such as MiraLAX or GoLYTELY, evacuate the bowel by washout without a significant fluid or electrolyte shift. Bisacodyl, available both as an oral preparation and a laxative, works by stimulating colonic peristalsis. Hyperosmotic preparations, such as the Fleet enema, draw water into the colon to achieve washout; however, caution must be used, as the risk of electrolyte abnormalities is greater with these methods of MBP.[29]

Controversy exists as to whether oral antibiotics should be administered as part of MBP.[30] A high bacterial load exists within the bowel lumen, leading some to administer oral antibiotics prior to surgeries involving entry into the bowel. Whereas some studies have demonstrated a significant reduction in surgical site infections (SSIs) with MBP that involves oral antibiotics,[31,32] other studies have not found a difference in SSI, although it was found that administration of oral antibiotics may lead to nausea, vomiting, and abdominal pain.[33] When used, a combination of neomycin with erythromycin base or metronidazole, known as the Nichols and Condon prep, is typically given the day prior to surgery.[30]

Antibiotics may be necessary prior to surgery and should be directed toward typical organisms at the planned surgical site. For example, a patient undergoing a procedure that involves entry into the gastrointestinal tract should receive prophylaxis against typical gastrointestinal organisms. Patients with planned entry into the urinary tract should receive urine culture-specific antibiotic coverage against culture-proven organisms if a urinary tract infection exists. For most procedures involving skin incisions, a first-generation cephalosporin is typically given prior to the procedure. To prevent infection-related complications postoperatively, it is recommended to administer preoperative antibiotics within 60 minutes of the start of the procedure.

Another important consideration in patients undergoing surgical procedures, especially in those with prolonged operative times, is for prophylaxis against venous thromboembolism. The use of pneumatic compression stockings (mechanical prophylaxis) placed on the calves of a patient prior to the start of the procedure is now fairly universal. Pharmacologic prophylaxis via the use of subcutaneous unfractionated heparin or low-molecular-weight heparin should be considered based on a variety of surgery and patient-related factors, including the length of surgery, type of surgery (cancer surgery vs. surgery for benign indications), and patient health status and comorbidities.

REFERENCES

1. Townsend C, Beauchamp R, Evers B, Mattox K. *Sabiston Textbook of Surgery*. Philadelphia: Saunders Elsevier; 2008.
2. Saklad MDM. Grading of patients for surgical procedures. *Anesthesiology*. 1941;2(3):281–284.
3. Goldman L, Caldera DL, Nussbaum SR, et al. Multifactorial index of cardiac risk in noncardiac surgical procedures. *New England Journal of Medicine*. 1977;297(16):845–850.
4. Linn BS, Linn MW, Wallen N. Evaluation of results of surgical procedures in the elderly. *Annals of Surgery*. 1982;195(1):90–96.
5. Finlayson EV, Birkmeyer JD. Operative mortality with elective surgery in older adults. *Effective Clinical Practice*. 2001;4(4):172–177.
6. Fleisher LA, Fleischmann KE, Auerbach AD, et al. 2014 ACC/AHA guideline on perioperative cardiovascular evaluation and management of patients undergoing noncardiac surgery: a report of the American College of Cardiology/American Heart Association Task Force on practice guidelines. *Journal of the American College of Cardiology*. 2014;64(22):e77–e137.
7. Eagle KA, Berger PB, Calkins H, et al. ACC/AHA guideline update for perioperative cardiovascular evaluation for noncardiac surgery—executive summary. A report of the American College of Cardiology/American Heart Association Task Force on Practice Guidelines (Committee to Update the 1996 Guidelines on Perioperative Cardiovascular Evaluation for Noncardiac Surgery). *Circulation*. 2002;105(10):1257–1267.
8. Hlatky MA, Boineau RE, Higginbotham MB, et al. A brief self-administered questionnaire to determine functional capacity (the Duke Activity Status Index). *American Journal of Cardiology*. 1989;64(10):651–654.
9. Girish M, Trayner Jr E, Dammann O, Pinto-Plata V, Celli B. Symptom-limited stair climbing as a predictor of postoperative cardiopulmonary complications after high-risk surgery. *Chest*. 2001;120(4):1147–1151.
10. Reilly DF, McNeely MJ, Doerner D, et al. Self-reported exercise tolerance and the risk of serious perioperative complications. *Archives of Internal Medicine*. 1999;159(18):2185–2192.
11. Djokovic JL, Hedley-Whyte J. Prediction of outcome of surgery and anesthesia in patients over 80. *Journal of the American Medical Association*. 1979;242(21):2301–2306.
12. Smetana GW. Preoperative pulmonary evaluation. *New England Journal of Medicine*. 1999;340(12):937–944.
13. Warner MA, Divertie MB, Tinker JH. Preoperative cessation of smoking and pulmonary complications in coronary artery bypass patients. *Anesthesiology*. 1984;60(4):380–383.
14. Hall JC, Tarala RA, Hall JL, Mander J. A multivariate analysis of the risk of pulmonary complications after laparotomy. *Chest*. 1991;99(4):923–927.
15. Smetana GW, Lawrence VA, Cornell JE. Preoperative pulmonary risk stratification for noncardiothoracic surgery: systematic review for the American College of Physicians. *Annals of Internal Medicine*. 2006;144(8):581–595.
16. Lawrence VA, Dhanda R, Hilsenbeck SG, Page CP. Risk of pulmonary complications after elective abdominal surgery. *Chest*. 1996;110(3):744–750.
17. Canet J, Gallart L, Gomar C, et al. Prediction of postoperative pulmonary complications in a population-based surgical cohort. *Anesthesiology*. 2010;113(6):1338–1350.
18. Halaszynski TM, Juda R, Silverman DG. Optimizing postoperative outcomes with efficient preoperative assessment and management. *Critical Care Medicine*. 2004;32(suppl 4):S76–S86.
19. Apfelbaum JL, Connis RT, Nickinovich DG, et al. Practice advisory for preanesthesia evaluation: an updated report by the American Society of Anesthesiologists Task Force on Preanesthesia Evaluation. *Anesthesiology*. 2012;116(3):522–538.
20. Wu WC, Schifftner TL, Henderson WG, et al. Preoperative hematocrit levels and postoperative outcomes in older patients undergoing noncardiac surgery. *Journal of the American Medical Association*. 2007;297(22):2481–2488.
21. Lee TH, Marcantonio ER, Mangione CM, et al. Derivation and prospective validation of a simple index for prediction of cardiac risk of major noncardiac surgery. *Circulation*. 1999;100(10):1043–1049.
22. Mathew A, Devereaux PJ, O'Hare A, et al. Chronic kidney disease and postoperative mortality: a systematic review and meta-analysis. *Kidney International*. 2008;73(9):1069–1081.
23. Leung AA, McAlister FA, Finlayson SR, Bates DW. Preoperative hypernatremia predicts increased perioperative morbidity and mortality. *American Journal of Medicine*. 2013;126(10):877–886.
24. Kirkham KR, Wijeysundera DN, Pendrith C, et al. Preoperative testing before low-risk surgical procedures. *Canadian Medical Association Journal*. 2015;187(11):E349–E358.
25. Goldman L, Caldera DL, Southwick FS, et al. Cardiac risk factors and complications in non-cardiac surgery. *Medicine*. 1978;57(4):357–370.
26. Carliner NH, Fisher ML, Plotnick GD, et al. Routine preoperative exercise testing in patients undergoing major noncardiac surgery. *American Journal of Cardiology*. 1985;56(1):51–58.
27. Joo HS, Wong J, Naik VN, Savoldelli GL. The value of screening preoperative chest x-rays: a systematic review. *Canadian Journal of Anaesthesia*. 2005;52(6):568–574.

28. Apfelbaum J, Caplan R, Connis R, Epstein B, Nickinovich D, Warner M. Practice guidelines for preoperative fasting and the use of pharmacologic agents to reduce the risk of pulmonary aspiration: application to healthy patients undergoing elective procedures. An updated report by the American Society of Anesthesiologists Committee on Standards and Practice Parameters. *Anesthesiology*. 2011;114(3):495–511.

29. Nelson DB, Barkun AN, Block KP, et al. Technology status evaluation report. Colonoscopy preparations. May 2001. *Gastrointestinal Endoscopy*. 2001;54(6):829–832.

30. Kumar AS, Kelleher DC, Sigle GW. Bowel preparation before elective surgery. *Clinics in Colon and Rectal Surgery*. 2013;26(3):146–152.

31. Cannon JA, Altom LK, Deierhoi RJ, et al. Preoperative oral antibiotics reduce surgical site infection following elective colorectal resections. *Diseases of the Colon and Rectum*. 2012;55(11):1160–1166.

32. Lewis RT. Oral versus systemic antibiotic prophylaxis in elective colon surgery: a randomized study and meta-analysis send a message from the 1990s. *Canadian Journal of Surgery*. 2002;45(3):173–180.

33. Espin-Basany E, Sanchez-Garcia JL, Lopez-Cano M, et al. Prospective, randomised study on antibiotic prophylaxis in colorectal surgery. Is it really necessary to use oral antibiotics? *International Journal of Colorectal Disease*. 2005;20(6):542–546.

CHAPTER 2

WELCOME TO THE OPERATIVE THEATER

WHY IS THERE AN OPERATING ROOM?

More than 44 million operative procedures are performed each year in the United States.[1] To optimize patient outcomes, standards of space, culture, and training have evolved over time. This is realized in the operating room (OR), where strict protocols for cleanliness, precision, and collaboration are required.

The modern-day OR has evolved from the historical operating theater, a nonsterile room where students and interested observers could watch a surgeon perform operative procedures. These rooms had tiered seating, either on the side or from a floor above with an open ceiling, allowing individuals to observe the surgeon. Today's OR emphasizes sterility and the prevention of infection by minimizing the presence of unnecessary personnel and managing airflow. The OR suite is a closed collection of rooms that allows for quick, easy access to supplies and instruments needed to perform an operation, the ability to anesthetize a patient in a controlled environment, and the opportunity to clean and sterilize previously used supplies for use in successive surgeries. It has rooms where operations are performed and includes dedicated spaces for equipment storage, instrument processing, and cleaning supplies, as well as managing real-time patient throughput, in each room.

Although the OR is uniquely suited to the performance of surgery, it is not equipped to conduct patient care either before or after an operation. Typically there is a preoperative holding area where patients await surgery. Here there is final assessment for surgery. Laboratory testing and previous physician exams are checked, the planned procedure and accompanying consent are reviewed, and a final assessment is performed to ensure an optimal outcome. Following surgery, patients are brought to the postoperative recovery room, where they awaken from surgery in a monitored setting. This is done to ensure stability in a safe environment before leaving the hospital or being transferred to an inpatient floor.

There are usually multiple entrances to the operative suite, including from the recovery room, preoperative holding area, and main OR entrance. Each provides necessary personal protective equipment (PPE) that should be donned prior to entering. Entrances are usually clearly marked, notifying individuals that they are entering a sterile area (Fig. 2.1). To assist in keeping the OR environment clean, as well as to avoid bringing contamination from the OR to areas outside of the hospital, clean scrub attire provided by the hospital is required. Street clothes are not permitted for concern of transporting pathogens from the community into the operative suite. For individuals entering the OR for a brief period, wearing a clean outer protective garment (typically referred to as a bunny suit) over one's clothing may be permitted (Fig. 2.2). The entrance to the OR usually also allows access to protective surgical attire such as caps and bouffants to cover hair, shoe covers to protect footwear, and surgical masks. When entering a room where surgery is being performed, a mask is necessary. Video 2.1 demonstrates appropriate operative room attire.

As mentioned previously, the operative suite is a highly specialized section of the hospital that houses many individual ORs, which usually are spacious, well-lit rooms with overhead surgical lighting, allowing an optimal environment for a surgeon to perform a procedure. Usually there are different OR setups to allow for different procedures. For example, whereas one OR may house a robotic surgical system, another may be set up with an operative microscope or C-arm machine for fluoroscopy. Each OR has numerous power outlets on different circuits to support instruments and supplies that require electricity. Some rooms may have dedicated specialized power outlets to serve power needs of equipment such as lasers. As patient temperature can affect outcomes, there must be a way to regulate the temperature and humidity inside the OR. Each room has centralized gases, including oxygen, as well as wall suction to aid in clearing smoke, blood, and other fluids from the operative field. In addition, each room should have surfaces that are easy to clean, thereby allowing for rapid patient turnover and the prevention of infection.

Although the overarching goal of the OR is to allow for surgical procedures to be performed in a clean,

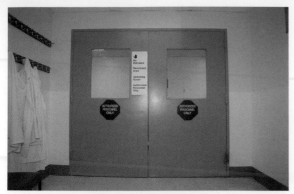

Fig. 2.1 Entrance to the OR

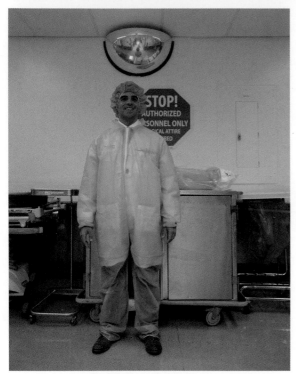

Fig. 2.2 Bunny suit garment

controlled environment, it also allows for education of students, surgical residents, and other physicians. There are often standing stools that allow surgeons and observers alike to gain a better view of a procedure. Modern ORs often have cameras and monitors that allow observers in the OR to view an operation without being immediately at the surgical table. Additionally, many ORs have the ability to record a surgery for later review.

BASIC COMPONENTS OF THE ROOM

Doors

The doorway to each OR, while oftentimes overlooked, serves a very important purpose in the room. The doors of the OR allow easy access by the surgeon and OR personnel while at the same time maintaining sterility within the room by minimizing traffic and airflow. It also allows a site to post signs, warning potential entrants in cases in which instruments are being used that require additional specialized PPE, such as a laser or C-arm. Construction is of many different materials, including wood or metal, depending on age and local fire codes (Fig. 2.3). There should be protection from radiation leakage built within the door in the event that x-ray is used in the room, including lead-containing windows if present. Doors can be hinged or sliding but should have a push handle or button to allow the scrubbed staff to enter the room without using their hands (Fig. 2.4).

The entrance to the OR should also be sufficiently wide to permit access to a patient bed and large OR support equipment. Entrance doors that are at least 6 feet wide typically allow enough space for most equipment. Dual-leaflet hinged doors permit a wide entranceway while minimizing the area required for door swing (Fig. 2.5).

Heating, Ventilating, and Air-Conditioning

Heating, ventilating, and air-conditioning systems, commonly referred to as HVAC, serve an integral role in the OR, as this is the route by which temperature and air quality is controlled. Additionally, maintaining proper humidity within the OR is important in reducing the risk of surgical infections. The Association of periOperative Registered Nurses (AORN) has constructed several guidelines with regard to the temperature, humidity, and airflow in perioperative areas (Table 2.1).[2] Suggested parameters for different areas of the perioperative suite, including unrestricted, semirestricted, and restricted areas are defined as:

Restrictive
- Invasive procedure room
- Operating room

Semirestricted
- Equipment and sterile supply storage
- Sterile processing area
- Sterile processing decontamination area

Semirestricted or Unrestricted
- Postanesthesia care unit

Unrestricted
- Endoscopy suite
- Locker room/administrative office/waiting room
- Pain clinic/procedure room
- Preoperative/postoperative patient care areas

Airflow within the OR, as defined by the number of air changes per hour, is an important part of minimizing environmental contamination and reducing surgical site infections. A minimum of 20 air changes per

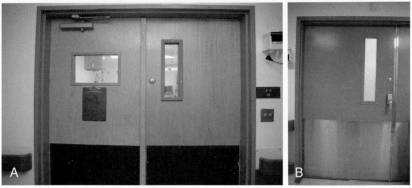

Fig. 2.3 OR door material. A. Wood. B. Metal.

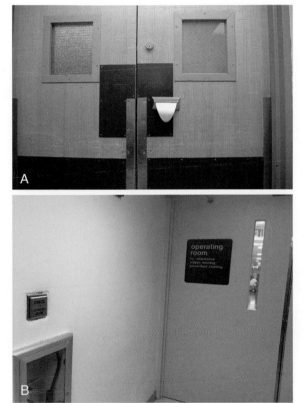

Fig. 2.4 OR door components. A. OR door with push handle. B. OR door with push button activation.

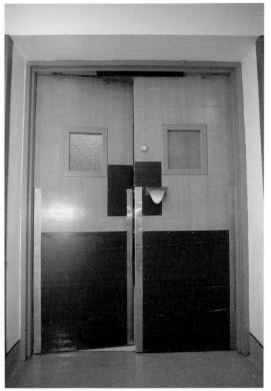

Fig. 2.5 Dual-leaflet doors

hour is recommended by the AORN for this purpose. By creating positive pressure within the room, air from the outside is prevented from moving into the sterile environment of the OR and is thought to impact on surgical site infections. For this reason, it is important to minimize opening the OR door during a procedure to maintain positive pressure.[3]

Lighting

Lighting within the OR is composed of three principal sources: main room lighting, overhead surgical lighting, and specialized purpose light sources. Main room lighting is the primary source of illuminating a room during preparation for a case, induction of anesthesia, and reversal of anesthesia after completing a procedure. During most open surgical procedures, the main room lights are left on to add illumination to the surgical field, as well as to provide lighting for assisting circulating and anesthesia personnel. These main room lights may be dimmed or turned off during endoscopic and laparoscopic procedures to enhance visualization of monitors. Main room lights, however, are poorly suited to provide direct illumination onto the surgical field and are therefore not used alone for this purpose during an open case.

Table 2.1 Airflow, Humidity, and Temperature of Perioperative Areas

	Airflow	Humidity	Temperature
Unrestricted	■ Related to the function performed in the area ■ Clean/sterile storage: positive ■ Soiled workroom/decontamination room: negative ■ Sterilizer equipment access: negative ■ Semirestricted corridor: no recommendations ■ Air changes per hour vary between 6 and 15 in procedure areas		■ 70–75°F (21–24°C)
Semirestricted	■ Related to the function performed in the area ■ Air changes per hour vary between 4 and 10	■ Clean/sterile storage: maximum 60% ■ Postanesthesia care unit, endoscopy and procedure rooms: 20–60%	■ Clean and sterile storage: 72–78°F (22–26°C) ■ Soiled workroom or decontamination room: 72–78°F (22–26°C)
Restricted	■ Positive pressure ■ 20 air changes per hour	■ Range of 20–60%	■ 68–75°F (20–24°C) Except for individual procedure needs

From AORN. Recommended practices for a safe environment of care, part II. Perioperative Standards and Recommended Practices. Denver, CO: AORN; 2014:e1–e25.

Overhead surgical lighting, by contrast, is used to illuminate the surgical field during a procedure. Surgical lighting should be sufficiently bright to provide adequate exposure to the surgical field. Typically two or more overhead surgical lights combine to form a surgical lighting system, which in concert works to provide different angles of bright illumination onto the surgical field. Overhead surgical lighting typically has a center handle onto which a sterile light cover is placed, allowing scrubbed individuals to manipulate them during a procedure. Additionally, there are usually multiple peripheral handles that are not sterile, giving nonscrubbed personnel access to lights for positioning (Fig. 2.6). Some surgical lighting is also equipped with a built-in camera, typically placed within the handle of the light, thereby allowing a procedure to be recorded or projected for better visualization of the surgical field for individuals not at the OR table.

Important characteristics of surgical lights include light intensity, light diameter, color rendition, and homogeneity. Light intensity, which describes the luminance of a surgical light, and light diameter should allow adequate visualization of the surgical field. Color rendition is the ability to distinguish the true color of tissues and should be as accurate as possible in surgical lighting. Homogeneity is the characteristic of a light that allows it to adequately illuminate a surgical field even when obstacles are placed between the light and field. Good light homogeneity is typically achieved via use of multiple surgical lights placed at different angles onto the field.[4]

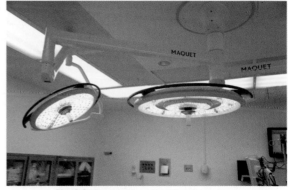

Fig. 2.6 Overhead surgical lighting system

Specialized light sources are used for a variety of indications. Most commonly, surgeons and assistants wear surgical headlights to better illuminate the operative field. Headlights typically allow the user to adjust the aperture through which light passes, therefore affecting the diameter of the light. With a constant light source, the intensity of light is inversely proportional to the diameter. For example, when the diameter of the light is increased, the intensity decreases. Conversely, when the diameter of the light is decreased, the intensity of the light increases. Headlights can be either battery powered or wired to a light source (Fig. 2.7).

Headlights allow a surgeon to illuminate deep surgical cavities, such as those encountered deep in the abdomen. The user must adjust the headlight to point in the direction of his vision prior to scrubbing and gowning into a procedure. Surgical headlights typically complement an overhead surgical lighting system and are rarely

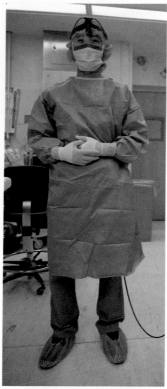

Fig. 2.7 Surgical headlight

used as the sole source of surgical lighting during a procedure. Endoscopes, such as laparoscopes, bronchoscopes, and cystoscopes, are instruments that plug into a light source to bring light inside a body cavity. These are usually coupled with a camera system that is used for visualization. Light intensity can be adjusted as dictated by the application.

Information Technology

Today's ORs are becoming increasingly technology driven. The movement from paper records to electronic health records within the greater healthcare system has driven the OR to adapt accordingly, with numerous advancements in technology being implemented in recent years. For example, most operative suites are now equipped with computers for charting the anesthesia record, inputting case information by the OR nurse, and display of relevant patient imaging studies. Endoscopic and laparoscopic towers are increasingly complex, usually equipped with high-definition monitors, and often allow for video recording capabilities. For this reason, the OR team now benefits from individuals trained in surgical technology support.

Additionally, patient-tracking and OR status-tracking services have increased in prevalence. Patient-tracking services allow OR personnel, surgeons,

anesthesiologists, and even patient family members to know the status and whereabouts of a patient undergoing surgery. For example, a monitor in the waiting room may allow a family member to track a patient's progress from the preoperative holding area, into the OR, and out of the OR and into the recovery room. OR-tracking services allow OR personnel and surgeons to track the status of an individual operating suite. These systems serve to replace the traditional OR status "board" and usually relay such information as when a patient enters the OR, when a case is in progress, when a case has completed and the drape is down, when the OR is being cleaned, and when the room is sterile and ready for the next patient (Fig. 2.8). Tracking is also available for large equipment and for disposables to help in managing/assessing the financial aspect of each case.

Power

Electrical supply to the operative suite is imperative. Control of anesthesia equipment and patient ventilators, lighting, and surgical equipment all reply on adequate, uninterrupted power to the OR. Additionally, numerous devices, such as lasers and x-ray equipment, require electrical power beyond what is provided by a standard 110-volt electrical supply outlet and may require a special outlet. For these reasons, several standards have been developed by the National Fire Protection Association (NFPA) for the delivery of power to the operative suite. For example, there should be at least 36 outlet receptacles to provide power; however, given the number of instruments in the OR that require electrical power, the number of outlets in each operative suite is often greater than this. In addition, given that fluids are used in some operative procedures, the OR is regarded as a "wet" location such that outlets are set up to provide protection against electric shock.[5]

Electrical outlets should be readily available at different sites in the OR. There should be at least one outlet on each wall, and often there are overhead ceiling outlets in towers that prevent multiple cords from running on the floor (Fig. 2.9). Although twist-lock connectors used to be popular for OR equipment to prevent their use outside of the OR and to minimize the risk of inadvertently having a plug disconnect, these have fallen out of use in most cases in favor of standard three-prong connectors (Fig. 2.10). Tape or special floor mats have been used to mitigate against the risk of power supply disconnect, as well as to prevent staff in the OR from tripping over wires (Fig. 2.11).

Given the severe impact a power failure could have on the course of an operation, ORs are required to have

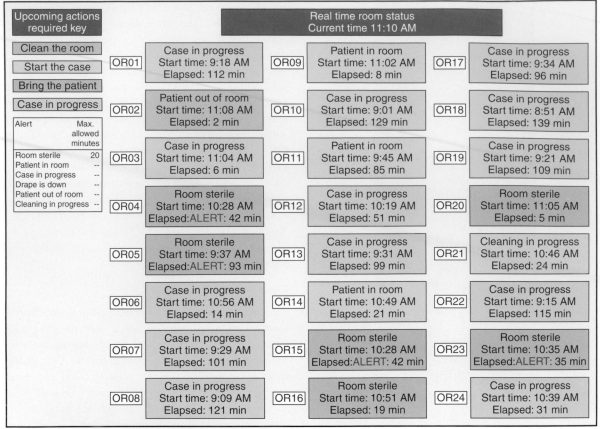

Upcoming actions required key		Real time room status Current time 11:10 AM	

Clean the room					
Start the case	OR01	Case in progress Start time: 9:18 AM Elapsed: 112 min	OR09	Patient in room Start time: 11:02 AM Elapsed: 8 min	OR17	Case in progress Start time: 9:34 AM Elapsed: 96 min
Bring the patient					
Case in progress	OR02	Patient out of room Start time: 11:08 AM Elapsed: 2 min	OR10	Case in progress Start time: 9:01 AM Elapsed: 129 min	OR18	Case in progress Start time: 8:51 AM Elapsed: 139 min

Alert	Max. allowed minutes
Room sterile	20
Patient in room	--
Case in progress	--
Drape is down	--
Patient out of room	--
Cleaning in progress	--

OR03	Case in progress Start time: 11:04 AM Elapsed: 6 min	OR11 Patient in room Start time: 9:45 AM Elapsed: 85 min	OR19 Case in progress Start time: 9:21 AM Elapsed: 109 min
OR04	Room sterile Start time: 10:28 AM Elapsed:ALERT: 42 min	OR12 Case in progress Start time: 10:19 AM Elapsed: 51 min	OR20 Room sterile Start time: 11:05 AM Elapsed: 5 min
OR05	Room sterile Start time: 9:37 AM Elapsed:ALERT: 93 min	OR13 Case in progress Start time: 9:31 AM Elapsed: 99 min	OR21 Cleaning in progress Start time: 10:46 AM Elapsed: 24 min
OR06	Case in progress Start time: 10:56 AM Elapsed: 14 min	OR14 Patient in room Start time: 10:49 AM Elapsed: 21 min	OR22 Case in progress Start time: 9:15 AM Elapsed: 115 min
OR07	Case in progress Start time: 9:29 AM Elapsed: 101 min	OR15 Room sterile Start time: 10:28 AM Elapsed:ALERT: 42 min	OR23 Room sterile Start time: 10:35 AM Elapsed:ALERT: 35 min
OR08	Case in progress Start time: 9:09 AM Elapsed: 121 min	OR16 Room sterile Start time: 10:51 AM Elapsed: 19 min	OR24 Case in progress Start time: 10:39 AM Elapsed: 31 min

Fig. 2.8 Electronic OR status board

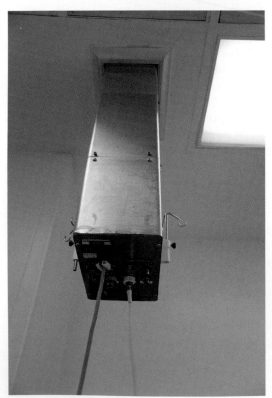

Fig. 2.9 Overhead ceiling outlet

emergency backup generators that can supply power to the OR in case of a power outage. This is usually in the form of a stand-alone power generator on-site at the hospital that is able to kick in immediately after power failure.[6]

OR Gases and Suction

Each OR typically has one or more locations with outlets for OR gases. This includes outlets that allow the delivery of gas as well as evacuation of gases, which can be located in wall outlets or in multipurpose ceiling columns that house electrical and other outlets (see Fig. 2.9). Rooms should have, at minimum, outlets for the delivery of medical air, oxygen, and nitrous gases in addition to vacuum outlets that permit the use of suction. The anesthesia team primarily utilizes the delivery of gases; however, suction is used by both anesthesia and surgical teams, and requires that multiple vacuum outlets be available in each OR.

Storage

The OR requires a large number of medical devices, disposable supplies, and instruments to be readily available. Some very specific implants and instruments are

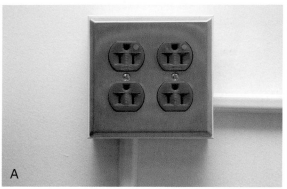
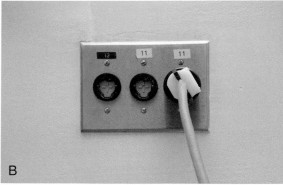

Fig. 2.10 Outlet connectors. A. Three-prong outlet connector. B. Twist-lock outlet connector.

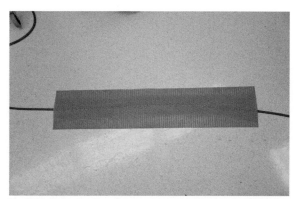

Fig. 2.11 Protective tape/floor mat to prevent power supply disconnect in the OR

not stored within the OR, and they are often ordered and brought in on a case-by-case basis. Most, however, are housed within the operating suite with specific, frequently used items within each OR itself. Some institutions have disposable equipment housed in a Pyxis system (CareFusion, San Diego, CA) and require entering a code to unlock a box containing the device. This helps with monitoring inventory and financial billing (Fig. 2.12).

Additional storage within the OR is also necessary for large equipment and less commonly used supplies. This allows each operative suite to remain clutter free while still allowing easy access to materials. Often a central supply storage area is used for this purpose. As per federal regulations, equipment should not be stored in hallways in the operative suite, as it may inhibit patient and equipment transport.

Some institutions use case carts to supply equipment to each case. These are large, rectangular closed carts that are stocked in a central supply core in the operative suite or elsewhere in the hospital. Disposable supplies are placed in each cart based on each case need and specific surgeon preference. The cart is then sent to the room with a checklist as needed. The nursing staff in the room references the checklist with what is in the

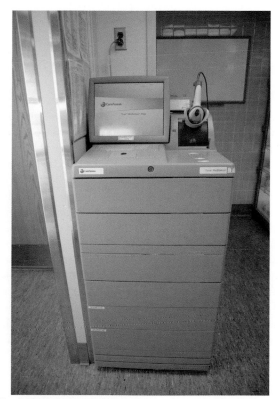

Fig. 2.12 Pyxis system for monitoring and cataloging disposable supplies

cart and may open additional supplies as required for the case.

Tables

OR tables and counters allow personnel the necessary working space during an operation. Although typically not sterile, general counter space is often utilized in the OR to fill out paperwork and organize nonsterile or unopened packages of instruments. Computers and other electronic equipment that is part of the OR may be found here as well. OR tables, in contrast, are usually draped with sterile coverings and allow the organization of sterile instruments and supplies. More complex operations may require two or more large tables to organize all of the instruments required for the operation.

OR tables are typically constructed of nonporous material such as stainless steel, which allows them to easily be cleaned after an operation. Two main OR tables are often utilized: the OR back table and the Mayo stand. The back table (Fig. 2.13) is a large table that allows for general organization of instruments and supplies away from the operative field. Scrub technicians pass instruments to and from the back table as they are needed during a procedure. The Mayo stand (Fig. 2.14), in contrast, is a height-adjustable table with a smaller working area that can be positioned over the patient table. This allows quick access to recently used and needed instruments and supplies. The back table and Mayo stand are often used together to organize instruments during a procedure.

Scrub Sink

Scrub sinks serve as general areas that allow surgeons and other personnel to disinfect their hands before donning sterile attire in the OR. They should be in close proximity to each OR. There is usually access to beta-dine- or chlorhexidine-containing scrub brushes, or scrub brushes on which betadine or chlorhexidine solution can be applied. Additionally, waterless antiseptic solution such as a chlorhexidine hand scrub is usually provided at scrub sinks (Fig. 2.15).

The flow of water at scrub sinks is usually activated and deactivated in one of two ways. Knee/foot-operated sinks allow for water control by tapping a pad on the front of the sink. Alternatively, some scrub sinks are equipped with an infrared sensor for water control such that when a sensor recognizes an individual's hands under the faucet, the flow of water is started. Additional features at some sinks include eye wash stations, digital timers, and knee/foot-operated soap dispensers (Fig. 2.16).

PERSONNEL

The complexity of performing surgery on another human being requires coordinated collaboration among a team of individuals to ensure success. Nurses, physicians, technicians, and administrative assistants are all essential personnel in the OR.

Nursing

Nurses serve the central organizational role in the OR. Whereas different surgeons and anesthesia teams may move in and out of different rooms on different days, nursing provides dedicated 24-hour full-time staffing to the space. Nursing personnel also oversee the entire operative suite. This includes managing the status board

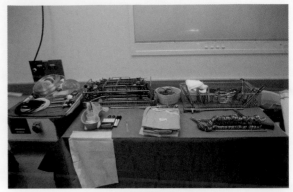

Fig. 2.13 OR back table

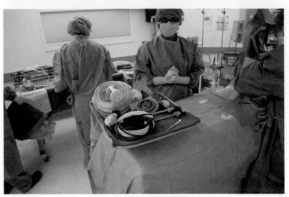

Fig. 2.14 Mayo stand

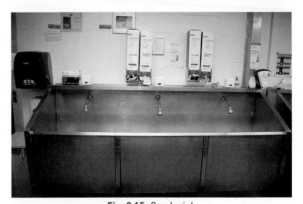

Fig. 2.15 Scrub sink

where efforts are coordinated to ensure that rooms are appropriately staffed and cases proceed on time. In each OR, nurses are responsible for coordinating equipment needs, documenting events, monitoring sterility, and assisting in the performance of the procedure. Numerous nurses usually participate in each individual case, including circulators, scrub technicians, and surgical assistants.

Circulators

OR circulators are typically registered nurses who are responsible for several roles during the course of

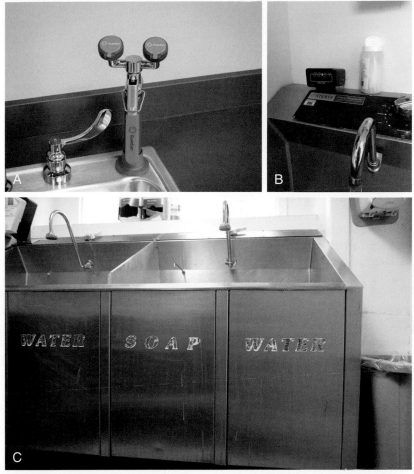

Fig. 2.16 Additional components to the scrub sink. A. Eye wash station. B. Digital timer. C. Knee-operated soap dispenser.

a procedure. First, circulators are in charge of making sure the room has all equipment available for an operation and that the room is set up appropriately. Circulators are often the ones who coordinate receiving a patient in the OR from the preoperative holding area. They verify both the identification of the patient and the intended surgery. The circulator accompanies the patient to the OR, introduces the patient to the staff, and helps position the patient on the table both before and after anesthesia is administered. Circulators also retrieve supplies needed throughout the procedure for both the surgeon and anesthesiologist. Circulators are responsible for handling specimens such as tissue, fluid, and blood, and making sure that they are correctly labeled and marked. In parallel, they chart in the OR record, including recording key time components such as time of induction of anesthesia, procedure start time, and time of incision; record supplies utilized during a surgery; and document unexpected events. Another key role of the OR circulator is to serve as an intermediary between the OR staff and the rest of the hospital. It is the circulator's responsibility to field calls into the OR,

call in other surgeons and personnel as needed, and alert the recovery room that a procedure has been completed.

Scrub Technicians

As opposed to OR circulators, scrub technicians (scrub techs), also known as surgical technicians or surgical technologists, do not need to be registered nurses. Although the role of a scrub technician may be fulfilled by a nurse, numerous degree programs exist in which individuals may become registered scrub technicians. Responsibilities of the scrub technician include setting up and organizing the sterile table for a procedure, handing instruments and supplies to the surgeon during the operation, and passing off instruments at the conclusion of a procedure. Scrub technicians observe the case and, as experienced individuals, can anticipate what instrument or supplies are needed before they are requested. They also keep track of what instruments were used during the case to avoid inadvertently leaving supplies in a patient. Scrub technicians request additional materials from the circulator when needed. Usually one scrub technician participates in each case;

however, in complex surgeries, there may be more than one.

Surgical Assistants

Surgical assistants are additional members of the OR team who assist the surgeon during surgery. Like scrub technicians, surgical assistants do not require a degree in nursing, although they often do have such credentials. Surgical assistants can do all of the work of scrub technicians but are also able to assist the surgeon more during the course of surgery. Particular roles of a surgical assistant can include help with retraction, suturing, suctioning, and other tasks as directed by the surgeon. As opposed to scrub technicians, who are required for nearly every operative case, surgical assistants may not be needed if other surgeons, physician assistants, or surgical residents are involved in a procedure.

Housekeeping and the Sterile Processing Department

Housekeepers and OR turnover staff serve a vital role in keeping the OR moving in an efficient and timely manner. At the conclusion of a procedure, housekeepers are responsible for cleaning the room and preparing it for subsequent surgeries. This includes clearing debris from the room, mopping the floors, wiping down and disinfecting the patient table, and sanitizing other surfaces in the OR. All visibly soiled surfaces must be cleaned in preparation for the next patient. In addition, disposable supplies such as ventilator tubing, intravenous (IV) tubing, and sequential compression device boots must be replaced. Performed in a timely manner, the OR can run as scheduled with the day's procedures.

The sterile processing department (SPD) is responsible for sterilizing instruments and reusable supplies at the completion of a procedure. As some instruments may take more than an hour to process and can be in limited supply in the OR, it is critical that the SPD work in an efficient manner to sterilize and prepare instruments for subsequent procedures. Although timely processing of instruments is important, the foremost responsibility of the SPD is to ensure sterility of processed instruments. If missed, an improperly sterilized instrument can cause delays in the OR while waiting for other instruments to arrive, or worse, could result in serious infection if used on a patient.

Anesthesia

Anesthesiologists, nurse anesthetists, and anesthesia residents are tasked at putting a patient to sleep, keeping a patient sedated during a procedure, and reversing anesthesia at the conclusion of surgery. Anesthesia can be administered in a variety of ways, with different levels of sedation, paralysis, and airway management

possible. The anesthesia team is also tasked with perioperative pain control, administering medications, and placing epidural catheters and nerve blocks. Prior to the start of surgery, the anesthesia team ensures adequate vascular access and often places IV lines as needed. They also set up physiologic monitoring as mandated by the case, which can include cardiac monitors, pulse oximeters, arterial lines, and central venous lines. The team monitors and cares for a patient during surgery, ensuring appropriate homeostasis and giving IV medications, fluids, and blood products, and alerts the surgical team to any unsafe circumstances. The anesthesia team also monitors and cares for patients immediately following a procedure.

Anesthesiologist

Anesthesiologists are physicians who have completed a residency in anesthesiology and are licensed to provide anesthesia. Just as the surgeon serves as the quarterback of the operative team, an anesthesiologist serves as the leader of the anesthesia team. The anesthesiologist determines the appropriate type and amount of anesthesia to give. An anesthesiologist may serve as the sole provider of anesthesia during the course of an operation, working one-to-one with a patient, or may supervise a team of nurse anesthetists and/or anesthesia residents.

Nurse Anesthetist

Certified registered nurse anesthetists (CRNAs) are registered nurses who are certified to provide anesthesia. After completing a degree program in nursing, those who wish to pursue a career as a CRNA must complete a master's degree in anesthesia or nursing with a post-master's certification in anesthesia. Additionally, they must work in an intensive care unit for a minimum of 1 year.[7] CRNAs are able to perform many of the same duties as an anesthesiologist, including placing lines, intubating, administering anesthetics, and extubating a patient. In numerous states CRNAs are permitted to practice independently; however, some states require that CRNAs be overseen by an anesthesiologist. The role of CRNAs in today's medical practice is rapidly increasing to allow more credentialed providers to administer anesthesia care.

Anesthesia Resident

Anesthesia residents are individuals in training to become licensed anesthesiologists. They can place lines, intubate, extubate, and monitor a patient during and after surgery under the supervision of a licensed anesthesiologist. Completion of an anesthesia residency requires a year of training in either a medical or surgical internship, followed by a 3-year training program in anesthesiology.

Surgical Team

The surgical team is tasked at carrying out the operative portion of the perioperative period. Several different surgical specialties exist, and each is uniquely suited to perform different procedures.

Attending Surgeon

Attending surgeons are the leaders of the surgical team. They are licensed to perform surgery in the discipline for which they have received training in residency. Attending surgeons typically see patients preoperatively in consultation in the office or on an emergent basis in the hospital or emergency department. They are tasked at deciding what surgical procedure to perform, how to perform that procedure, and following patients through their recovery postoperatively.

Attending surgeons direct the rest of the surgical team, including assistants, surgical technicians, and circulators throughout the course of an operation. They decide what instruments are necessary to complete a procedure, what suture material is best suited for individual tissues and purposes, and how to best approach a surgical case. The attending surgeon typically also supervises and teaches fellows, residents, medical students, and other assistants in the OR during a procedure.

Assistant Surgeon

Surgical assistants can be any number of individuals. Many larger procedures benefit from multiple assistants who may contribute by suturing, retracting, cutting, or other roles. In academic institutions, surgical residents acting under the direction of an attending surgeon may greatly contribute to a procedure. As discussed previously, surgical assistants, including those credentialed as stand-alone surgical assistants, nursing surgical assistants, and physician assistants also can fulfill this role.

Surgical Resident

Surgical residents have completed medical school and are currently participating in residency training in a particular surgical field. Surgical residencies vary in length but typically entail between 4 and 6 years of postgraduate medical training, including a 1- or 2-year internship prior to commencing residency training. Residents usually take an active role in performing surgical procedures under the direction of an attending surgeon. It is during this time as a surgical resident that the necessary knowledge and skill is acquired to act alone as an attending surgeon.

REFERENCES

1. Hall MJ, DeFrances CJ, Williams SN, Golosinskiy A, Schwartzman A. National Hospital Discharge Survey: 2007 summary. *National Health Statistics Reports*. 2010;(29):1–20, 24.
2. Recommended practices for a safe environment of care, part II. *Perioperative Standards and Recommended Practices*. Denver, CO: AORN; 2014:e1–e25.
3. Bartley JM, Olmsted RN, Haas J. Current views of health care design and construction: practical implications for safer, cleaner environments. *American Journal of Infection Control*. 2010;38(5 suppl 1):S1–S12.
4. IEC. Medical electrical equipment—part 2-41: particular requirements for the basic safety and essential performance of surgical luminaires and luminaires for diagnosis. IEC 60601-2-41:2009; 2009.
5. NFPA. *NFPA 99: Health Care Facilities Handbook*. Washington, DC: NFPA; 2005.
6. Helfman S. *Electrical service. Operating Room Design Manual*. Washington, DC: American Society of Anesthesiologists; 2010:69–75.
7. Nagelhout JJ, Elisha S, Plaus K. *Nurse Anesthesia*. St. Louis, MO: Elsevier Health Sciences; 2013.

CHAPTER 3
SCRUBBING AND STAYING STERILE

BASICS OF THE STERILE ENVIRONMENT

Historically, infection was the biggest cause of morbidity and mortality following a surgical procedure. Discoveries in the late 1800s provided the impetus and means to eliminate bacteria both from wounds and the operating room (OR) environment. Today's ORs are set up to provide as clean an environment as possible, with the objective of creating operative field sterility, which is defined as the absence of all viable organisms.

In the OR, the floor, walls, lights, ceilings, and other equipment are maintained to be very clean; however, current practicalities make it such that there are still microbes in the environment. It is possible, though, to create a near-sterile environment in the immediate operative space, inclusive of drapes used to cover the patient, the back table used to organize instruments, garments worn by individuals at the OR table, and the exposed operative site on the patient.

Great care is taken to ensure that the OR is meticulously cleaned and disinfected prior to a patient entering the room. There are a variety of ways in which this is accomplished. Basic cleaning involves removing all visible contaminants from a surface. In between cases, a cleaning crew removes all debris from the previous operation, including blood and body fluids from surfaces and equipment that are to remain in the room. All visible blood and bodily fluids from previous cases must be thoroughly removed, usually with a combination of soap and water followed by an alcohol-based germicidal disinfecting solution. High-level disinfection is a process that kills all viable microorganisms with the exception of large numbers of bacterial spores, whereas sterilization kills all microorganisms and spores.[1] Sterilization, therefore, provides the greatest assurance that instrumentation and surgical equipment are free of viable organisms for use in surgical procedures.

Once the room is cleaned, the nursing team begins to bring needed equipment into the OR. The OR bed is covered with a clean sheet, as are arm boards that are placed on either side to support the patient's arms during induction of anesthesia. Safety straps are placed on the table to secure the patient to the table. An anesthesia technician who has removed debris from the anesthesia area sets up new ventilation tubing and intravenous (IV) lines.

It is not practical to sterilize the entire room, and therefore a microenvironment surrounding the operative site is created. After the room has been deemed "clean," the sterile field is created. The scrub nurse/technician begins preparing the back table of instruments and disposable supplies necessary for the surgery. This includes patient drapes and gowns that will be worn by individuals at the operating table.

It is the responsibility of all individuals in the OR to maintain standards and keep the sterile field intact at all times. Once a patient is positioned, he or she is prepped with a solution such as chlorhexidine or iodine to provide surgical site disinfection and then covered with a sterile drape to isolate the operative site (Fig. 3.1). The sterile field typically includes a covered back table, on which instruments that may be used during the case are organized, and a Mayo table, which is positioned over the patient and holds instruments and disposable supplies that are actively being used at any given point in the case. There can also be stands with sterile solutions, as well as larger instruments (e.g., C-arms), robots, and microscopes that are covered with plastic drapes while in the operative field. Only scrubbed and gowned personnel such as the surgeon, scrub technician, and assistants are permitted to touch anything in this area to ensure ongoing sterility. It is imperative that nonscrubbed individuals refrain from touching any part of the sterile field during a procedure and that scrubbed personnel minimize their movement away from the sterile field, as this increases the possibility of contamination.

Today, disposable drapes, gowns, and covers usually mark the sterile environment. These are of a uniform color to define the sterile area, usually light blue or green. Washable cloth gowns and drapes have traditionally been used, but in many institutions these

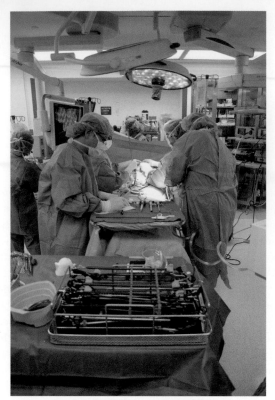

Fig. 3.1 Sterile field at patient bedside

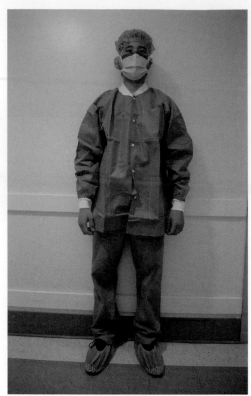

Fig. 3.2 OR attire including OR jacket

have been replaced in favor of disposable supplies. Although the overall cost of single-use materials in the OR is higher than reusable materials, the cost-benefit ratio of single-use supplies has led to their preferential use, as they minimize the risk of infection and are easily handled.[2]

It is important that all individuals in the OR, from the time the room is considered sterile until the end of the procedure, don appropriate scrub attire. This includes surgical scrubs, a head covering such as a bouffant, and a surgical mask. Shoe coverings are required if footwear from outside the OR environment is worn. Individuals in the OR who are not scrubbed should also minimize the amount of uncovered skin and hair by wearing an OR jacket (Fig. 3.2). Donning appropriate OR attire minimizes the transfer of hair, dust, and microorganisms from personnel within the OR to the sterile field.

Limiting traffic in the OR also helps minimize contamination of the sterile field. The greater the number of individuals in the room during a procedure, the greater the risk of introducing microorganisms. Each time the OR doors are opened, positive pressure within the room is reduced, inhibiting movement of dust, lint, and microbes away from the sterile field as intended. It is therefore important to limit the number

of individuals entering the OR who do not contribute to the procedure.

The OR can be a place of stress and intimidation, especially for students, trainees, and new employees. However, it is the role of all individuals in the OR to immediately call to attention any unsafe situations, including breaks in sterility. This "surgical conscience" creates the safest environment not only for the patient but also for the healthcare workers caring for the patient. It also allows any identified problems to be corrected as quickly and efficiently as possible to prevent further contamination of the field.

THE STERILE FIELD

Minimizing the risk of surgical site infection (SSI) begins with strict adherence to maintaining sterility during a procedure. Before the patient even enters the room, there are several measures that can be taken to prevent SSI. This is initiated by thoroughly cleaning the OR to clear debris and contamination from prior procedures. A meticulous process of sterilizing instruments in a separate processing area occurs to ensure the lowest risk of their contamination. After the OR has been cleaned from the previous procedure, traffic in the room should be minimized to prevent loss of positive

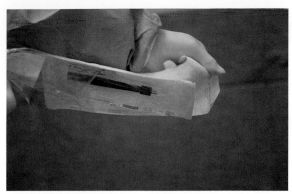

Fig. 3.3 Opening a peel-packed instrument in a sterile manner

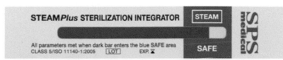

Fig. 3.4 Autoclave indicator demonstrating appropriate instrument processing during sterilization. Used with permission from SPSmedical Supply Corp.

pressure in the room and to prevent the introduction of microbes into the OR.

When preparing the sterile back table, several considerations are taken. First, all peel-packed instruments and supplies should be opened so that their contents are allowed to fall onto the sterile surface (Fig. 3.3), or should allow a scrubbed individual to withdraw the contents without touching the nonsterile outside of the packaging. The nonsterile individual who is opening the package, by the same manner, should refrain from touching the inside of the sterile package. Disposable supplies often have an expiration date that should be checked prior to use during a procedure. For instruments that have been reprocessed, packaging should be checked to ensure that there are no holes that would result in contamination. Many instruments that have been processed in an autoclave also contain an indicator within the packaging that signifies that it has been appropriately processed (Fig. 3.4). This indicator should be checked each time a new instrument is opened to ensure that it has been adequately sterilized. An additional consideration that is often overlooked is the preparation of the sterile field as close as possible to the start of the procedure. By reducing the amount of time a sterile field is open prior to its use, the potential for contamination by staff, the patient, and ambient particles such as dust is minimized.

After the patient has been anesthetized, IV and other lines have been placed, and the patient has been positioned and secured to the table, skin shaving

should be performed if indicated. At this time, the surgical site is prepared via use of a disinfecting solution, commonly a chlorhexidine- or betadine-containing solution. The operative field should be prepped so that the planned site of the incision is prepared first, with preparation of the surrounding skin following. The skin is commonly prepared in concentric circles extending outward from the planned incision site (Video 3.1). It is important to allow the skin prep adequate time to dry prior to placing the sterile drapes on the patient. This allows for adequate microbial kill by the skin prep solution and prevents fires and skin burn injury via the use of electrocautery and other electricity-generating surgical instruments. In most cases, allowing the skin prep to dry for 3 minutes is sufficient.

When placing sterile drapes, it is important to minimize their movement in the environment as much as possible. Excessive movement of draping material causes ambient environmental contaminants such as dust and lint to move, possibly contaminating the sterile field. It is also important to minimize air movement and contact at the surgical site itself as much as possible. As such, drapes should be placed on the patient with the first contact and drape opening at the surgical site, then expanded to the periphery (Fig. 3.5). After applying the patient drape, and especially when using draping material with adhesive edges, the drape should not be moved. By moving the drape, this allows material previously over an unprepared area to contact a sterilized area of the patient's skin, thus contaminating that region. Towel clips and staples may also been used to fix drapes into position.

Once the patient drape has been applied, surgical instruments with cables and tubing should be secured to the field to prevent contact with nonsterile individuals and objects in the OR (Fig. 3.6). This should be done with nonperforating instruments, such as Allis clamps (see Chapter 5). The use of perforating devices creates holes in the drapes that cause a break in the sterile protective barrier of the drape. Additionally, certain instruments, such as fluoroscopy units and ultrasound probes, are unable to undergo sterilization and should be covered with sterile drapes prior to their use during a procedure (Fig. 3.7).

It is important to minimize movements directly around the field by both scrubbed individuals and nonsterile personnel in the OR. Once the sterile field has been established, it is imperative that breaks in sterility be recognized immediately and corrected appropriately. This may be by any number of measures, including replacing contaminated drapes, gloves, and gowns, or by placing a sterile covering over an area with a break in sterility.

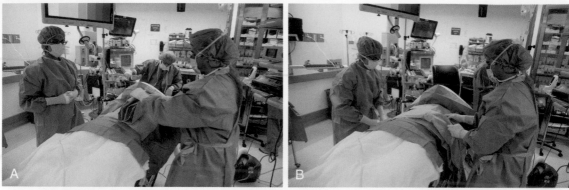

Fig. 3.5 Correct placement of patient drape. A. Drape first placed at the surgical site. B. Drape unfolded to the periphery.

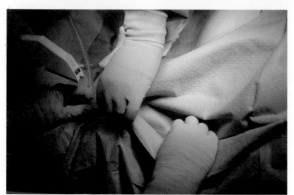

Fig. 3.6 Securing cables and tubing to the sterile field

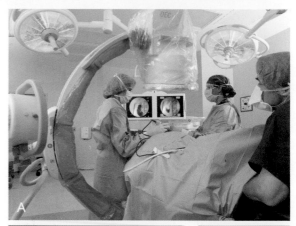

SCRUBBING

The surgical hand scrub is an integral part of preventing SSI (Video 3.2). Although sterile gloves and gowns are used, very small and unnoticeable perforations and breaches in protective gear can contaminate the field. By performing an adequate surgical scrub, dirt and debris are removed from the hands, forearms, and periungual and subungual areas. Additionally, the inoculum of microorganisms within these areas is greatly reduced, and regrowth is inhibited.[3]

Two methods of performing a surgical hand scrub have generally been employed. In the first (traditional) method, water is used to wet the surface of the hands and forearms, and then a brush with an alcohol or iodine-containing solution is used to mechanically dislodge contaminants and chemically disinfect the hands and forearms. The second method utilizes an alcohol-based solution, which is rubbed over the surface of the hands and forearms. In this method, water is not first employed (although a prewash with soap and water should be performed to remove dirt), and a brush is not used to apply the solution. These two methods of surgical hand antisepsis have been found to be comparable at eradicating microorganisms on the hands and forearms, although the waterless, brushless technique is faster and has improved compliance with handwashing

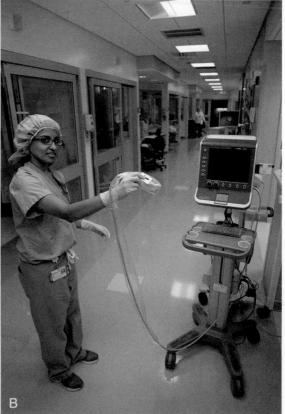

Fig. 3.7 Draping used for special instruments. A. Fluoroscopy unit with sterile drape applied. B. Ultrasound probe with sterile drape applied.

among surgeons.[4] Both techniques have been approved for performing the first scrub of the day in addition to subsequent scrubs.

It is important to remove all rings, bracelets, watches, and other jewelry from the hands prior to initiating a surgical scrub. This allows the areas under these items to be thoroughly cleaned and eliminates them as a source of microorganisms. Fingernails should be kept neat and clean, and trimmed to within ¼ inch in length. Although it may be advisable to refrain from wearing nail polish, it is important to only wear nail polish that has been placed within the previous 4 days and is not chipped or cracked. Freshly applied nail polish has not been shown to increase the inoculum of microorganisms as compared to native fingernails; however, worn, cracked, and chipped nail polish does increase the inoculum.[5,6] Artificial fingernails should never be worn, as they have been linked to SSIs. Additionally, artificial fingernails increase the risk of perforations in surgical gloves, presenting a risk to both the patient and healthcare worker.[7,8]

Prior to carrying out a surgical scrub, a prewash with soap and water should be performed. This removes all visible dirt and debris from the hands and forearms but does not considerably reduce the inoculum of microorganisms on the skin. During the prewash, subungual and periungual areas should be cleaned with a specialized nail-cleaning tool to remove dirt and debris from underneath and around the fingernails (Fig. 3.8). The hands should then be dried with a clean towel prior to initiating the surgical hand scrub.

The surgical scrub itself, both with a waterless, brushless solution or by the traditional method, begins at the tips of the fingers, progresses to the hands, and then proceeds to a point on the arms approximately 2 inches above the elbows. The surface of each individual finger should be thoroughly scrubbed multiple times. It is important to ensure that creases in the fingers and palms of the hands, as well as the areas between the fingers, are adequately cleansed. At all times during a traditional scrub, the hands should be kept above the level of the elbows, ensuring that previously cleaned areas are not contaminated with dirty water as it flows from unclean areas.

When performing a waterless, brushless scrub, the recommended amount of solution is dispensed into the palm of one hand. The fingers of the opposite hand are then dipped into this solution and worked into the subungual areas. The same process is applied to the subungual areas of the opposite hand. The remaining solution is then applied to all surfaces of the hands and arms to a point 2 inches above the elbows. It is advisable to then reapply the solution only to the hands after a full application to the arms. It is also important to ensure

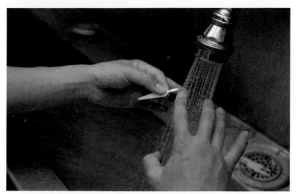

Fig. 3.8 Nail-cleaning tool used to remove dirt and debris from periungual and subungual areas

that the solution has dried prior to donning a surgical gown and gloves.

When performing a traditional scrub, either an iodine-based solution or chlorhexidine-based solution may be used. The brush containing the solution should be used to thoroughly scrub all surfaces of the fingers, hands, and forearms. To adequately perform a traditional scrub, two methods may be used to ensure a complete scrub. The timed scrub method utilizes a timer, typically set to 3 minutes or longer, to ensure that an adequate amount of time has been spent on a surgical scrub. This is in contrast to the counted stroke method, in which an individual counts the number of scrub strokes on each skin surface. Using the counted stroke method, each of the four surfaces of the fingers and arms (front, back, and either side) are scrubbed a set number of times. Different institutions use different protocols for the counted stroke method, but generally 10 or more strokes per surface are performed.

After completing a surgical scrub, it is important to prevent contaminating oneself prior to donning a surgical gown and gloves. To prevent dirty water from contaminating recently scrubbed hands and arms, the hands and arms should be held away from the body, above the waist, and with the hands above the elbows (Fig. 3.9). The scrubbed individual should not use his hands to open the OR door. To enter, doors are usually equipped with push buttons or handles that allow the individual to use his back to open the door. As such, a scrubbed individual should not touch any other surfaces with his hands or forearms.

DONNING A GOWN AND GLOVES

After performing a surgical scrub, there are two ways to don a gown and gloves without compromising the sterility of the sterile back table, patient drapes, and oneself. The first (assisted) method allows a scrub tech or other individual who is already scrubbed to assist in donning

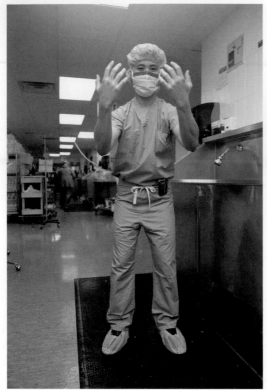

Fig. 3.9 Proper posture to prevent contaminating recently scrubbed hands and arms

the gown and gloves. The second method requires the individual to self-gown and self-glove. If the individual has performed a traditional scrub prior to donning a gown and gloves, she should first dry her hands with a sterile towel. Holding the towel in the corner with one hand, it is used to dry all surfaces of the other hand and arm, starting with the fingers and progressing to the elbow. Grasping the towel with the other hand in a dry corner, the process is then repeated to dry the other hand and arm. If an alcohol-based dry solution has been used to perform the scrub, it is not necessary to dry the hands.

To don a gown and gloves via the assisted method, the scrub tech fully opens the gown, being mindful of the surroundings so as to not contaminate the gown by touching nonsterile objects. The gown is held on the outside just above the sleeves. The scrubbed individual keeps his arms outstretched, and the scrub tech places the gown sleeves over the individual's arms. A nonsterile assistant should then tie the back of the gown and close the neck, securing the gown around the individual. At this point, the scrub tech should assist in placing sterile gloves. It is important to keep one's hands within the cuff of the gown prior to glove placement. As the gloves are placed, the individual's hands come through the gown cuff and into the gloves. It is customary to start by placing the

glove on the right hand, followed by the left. Once the right hand has been gloved, the individual can aid in placing the left glove by holding the glove open with his right hand.

Gowns additionally have an outside tie to help cover the back where the assistant first tied the gown closed. There is usually a pull-away paper or knot in front of the gown that secures the two ends of this outer tie during the gowning process. The paper or tie on the long end is handed to another sterile individual. Alternatively, a nonsterile individual can assist by grasping only the edge of the paper. While holding the shorter end of the tie, the gowning individual spins in a counterclockwise direction and then releases the long end of the tie from the paper hold by pulling on it. The short and long ends are then tied together by the scrubbed individual to secure the knot (Video 3.3).

To self-don a gown and gloves, the individual first picks up the gown by the folded inner surface, being careful not to touch surrounding sterile drapes and equipment. Both arms are then placed through the armholes, allowing the gown to fall open. At this point, a nonsterile assistant secures the back of the gown as in the assisted gowning and gloving method. The hands are kept within the cuff of the gown, and the sleeve is used as a mitten. The unopened right glove is picked up with the left hand and placed over the cuff of the right hand, allowing the hand to come through the cuff of the gown as it enters the glove. The cuff of the right glove is left unferruled. With the gloved right hand, the left glove is picked up by placing the fingers of the right hand between the inverted cuff of the left glove and the outer surface of the glove. The left glove is then placed over the cuff of the left gown sleeve, again allowing the left hand to come through the cuff of the gown as it enters the glove. With the gloved left hand, the right glove cuff is fully brought over the right gown cuff, then the same procedure is repeated on the left side. As with the assisted method, the outer tie of the gown is secured with the aid of an assistant (Video 3.4).

It is important to understand several nuances once one is gowned. First, the entire gown is not considered sterile. The sides of the gown and the back are deemed nonsterile due to the assistance provided by others in placing the gown, as well as the inability to monitor them fully for contamination during a procedure. Only the front of the gown from the level of the patient drapes to the chest is considered a sterile region. Additionally, the sleeves of the gown are considered sterile from the gloved hand to a point 2 inches above the elbow (Fig. 3.10). The cuff of the gown, however, is not considered sterile once placed. As such, the glove must cover the gown cuff.

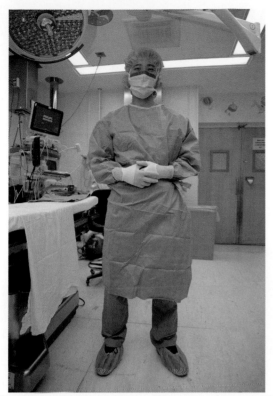

Fig. 3.10 Gowned individual demonstrating areas of gown sterility

It is also important to select a gown of appropriate size for each individual. Gowns that are too large and bulky permit contamination, as the redundant areas of the gown can come into contact with nonsterile equipment and individuals in the environment. Conversely, gowns that are too small for an individual may not close completely in the back, may tear during the procedure, or may allow the nonsterile cuff of the gown to become exposed from the gloves due to short sleeves.

In general, surgical gloves are constructed of either latex or latex-free material. It is important to select latex-free gloves for patients or healthcare workers with a latex allergy. Many institutions now preferentially recommend the use of latex-free gloves to eliminate the possibility of adverse reactions due to an unknown or undisclosed latex allergy.

It is also advisable to don two pairs of gloves during a surgical procedure. By wearing two pairs of gloves, thermal injury from surgical equipment is reduced, contamination of the operative field is prevented, and the chance of a needlestick injury and contracting a bloodborne illness is reduced.[9] The outer pair of gloves typically is fitted to the individual's hand size, whereas the inner pair of gloves is selected to be ½ size larger. The smaller outer glove prevents slippage of the inner glove. More importantly, however, it is imperative to

select a combination of gloves that is comfortable to the wearer.

MAINTAINING STERILITY

Maintaining sterility is the responsibility of all individuals in the OR, including both those who are scrubbed and those who are nonsterile. In particular, nonsterile individuals should refrain from coming too close to the sterile field or to individuals who are scrubbed into the procedure. It is also their responsibility to ensure that nonsterile equipment be kept at a safe distance from the operative field to prevent contact with sterile drapes.

For those who are scrubbed at the sterile field, there are several considerations to maintain sterility. Movement away from the sterile field should be minimized, as this increases the chance of contact with nonsterile individuals and equipment. It also allows for the movement of dust and debris that can subsequently come in contact with the sterile field. Changing levels, such as moving from a sitting to a standing position or vice versa, also increases the likelihood of contamination of the sterile field and thus should be minimized or avoided altogether. To this end, a scrubbed individual should never turn her back to the sterile field, as this greatly increases the chance of contact between the nonsterile back of the gown and the sterile field.

It is also important to maintain the sterility of the surgical gown. As such, arms and hands should always be kept above the waist when not at the sterile field. Placing one's hands over the front of the gown, oftentimes with interlocking fingers, is an easy way to prevent contamination of the arms and hands. When at the patient bedside and in the sterile field, arms and hands should always be kept above the level of the patient table and in the sterile field. Folding one's arms with the hands in the armpits should be discouraged, as the armpit is an area of friction and perspiration and thus is not sterile.

When it is necessary to move at the sterile field, movement should be accomplished as efficiently and with as little extraneous movements as possible. In cases in which two scrubbed individuals need to switch positions, they should turn either back-to-back or front-to-front while maintaining a safe distance from one another (Fig. 3.11). It is also important not to allow one individual to turn his back to the sterile field; therefore, when in close proximity to the sterile field, it is advised to turn back-to-back.

When passing instruments and supplies to surgeons and assistants, the instruments should always remain within the sterile field. Passing instruments around the back of other scrubbed individual risks contamination

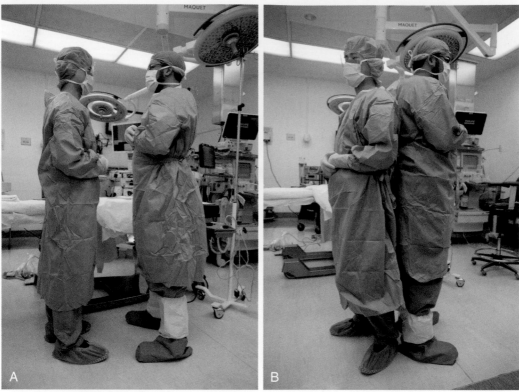

Fig. 3.11 Coordinated turning between two scrubbed individuals. A. Front-to-front. B. Back-to-back.

of both the instrument and the person passing the instrument. Additionally, when delivering instruments and supplies to the sterile field, such as when opening peel-packed instruments or disposable supplies, nonsterile individuals and packaging should not extend over the sterile field. Lightweight supplies may be dropped onto the sterile field; however, to prevent contamination, it is preferred that a scrub tech or other scrubbed individual receive the instrument or supply by removing it from the packaging.

DOFFING A GOWN AND GLOVES

While doffing (removing) a gown and gloves may seem intuitive, it is important to do so properly and carefully to prevent inadvertent exposure of healthcare workers to blood and bodily fluids that may be on these protective garments. If wearing two pairs of gloves, the outer pair may carefully be removed by pulling at the cuff and inverting the glove. This allows the clean inner pair of gloves to be used to remove the rest of the surgical gown. While still wearing at least one pair of surgical gloves, the outer gown tie should be untied or broken to release it. For reusable gowns, an assistant can then untie the back of the gown. For paper gowns, the gown is grasped at the sides with both hands, and with a firm pulling motion, the back inner tie is broken. At this

point the gown should be inverted, leaving the dirty outside of the gown facing inside, and the inside of the gown outside. The sleeves of the gown are accordingly inverted as well. Without touching one's skin, the gloves are removed along with the gown and inverted as well. At this point the inverted gown and gloves should be rolled together to keep the dirty outside facing in and placed in the proper trash receptacle. If a perforation is recognized after removing the surgical attire, the individual should immediately cleanse her hands and arms, then make sure there has not been an injury to the healthcare worker.

If a scrubbed individual's gown becomes contaminated during the course of a procedure, the gown and gloves should be removed (Video 3.5) and the individual should rescrub and don a gown and gloves. Alternatively, if an individual's glove becomes contaminated, the circulator or another nonscrubbed individual should aid in removing the glove by pulling near the cuff of the glove on the outside and inverting the glove. Care should be taken not to touch the scrubbed individual's hands, gown, or inner pair of gloves. At this point, another pair of sterile gloves can be donned without the need to perform a repeat scrub. Alternatively, if the sleeve of a gown becomes contaminated, sterile sleeve covers can be placed over the gown to protect sterility.

REFERENCES

1. Wallace CA. New developments in disinfection and sterilization. *American Journal of Infection Control.* 2016;44(suppl 5):e23–e27.
2. Baykasoglu A, Dereli T, Yilankirkan N. Application of cost/benefit analysis for surgical gown and drape selection: a case study. *American Journal of Infection Control.* 2009;37(3):215–226.
3. Tanner J, Dumville JC, Norman G, Fortnam M. Surgical hand antisepsis to reduce surgical site infection. *Cochrane Database of Systematic Reviews.* 2016;(1):CD004288.
4. Parienti JJ, Thibon P, Heller R, et al. Hand-rubbing with an aqueous alcoholic solution vs traditional surgical hand-scrubbing and 30-day surgical site infection rates: a randomized equivalence study. *Journal of the American Medical Association.* 2002;288(6):722–727.
5. Boyce JM, Pittet D. Guideline for hand hygiene in health-care settings. Recommendations of the Healthcare Infection Control Practices Advisory Committee and the HICPAC/SHEA/APIC/IDSA Hand Hygiene Task Force. Society for Healthcare Epidemiology of America/Association for Professionals in Infection Control/Infectious Diseases Society of America. *MMWR Recommendations and Reports.* 2002;51(RR-16):1–45. quiz CE1–4.
6. Wynd CA, Samstag DE, Lapp AM. Bacterial carriage on the fingernails of OR nurses. *AORN Journal.* 1994;60(5):796. 799–805.
7. Parry MF, Grant B, Yukna M, et al. Candida osteomyelitis and diskitis after spinal surgery: an outbreak that implicates artificial nail use. *Clinical Infectious Diseases.* 2001;32(3):352–357.
8. Toles A. Artificial nails: are they putting patients at risk? A review of the research. *Journal of Pediatric Oncology Nursing.* 2002;19(5):164–171.
9. Matta H, Thompson AM, Rainey JB. Does wearing two pairs of gloves protect operating theatre staff from skin contamination? *British Medical Journal (Clinical Research Ed.).* 1988;297(6648):597–598.

CHAPTER 4

PATIENT POSITIONING AND PREPPING

A patient may either walk, ride a wheelchair, or be rolled on a stretcher into the operating room (OR), depending both on individual hospital protocol and patient status/ability. Once the patient is in the OR, all staff members are prepared to increase the pace of activity. The various team members work independently, yet in concert, to initiate the start of surgery. There is comprehensive communication among team members at all times.

The first step, aided by the patient's participation, is verification of patient identity and the procedure to be performed. This "sign-in" procedure allows the patient to be a part of the process, confirming the procedure and laterality, and serving to prevent surgical errors. The patient is then positioned on the OR table, and the anesthesia team applies monitoring equipment such as a blood pressure (BP) cuff, telemetry leads, and a pulse oximeter.

The patient may or may not have had intravenous (IV) access initiated in the preoperative holding area prior to entering the OR. Anesthesia is responsible for assessing IV access and ensuring that there is adequate access to administer medications, blood, and IV fluids to maintain homeostasis during the procedure. Should a patient have not entered the OR with IV access, the anesthesia team obtains access at this time. Complex operations may require the anesthesia team to place multiple lines for both vascular access and more sophisticated monitoring.

The nursing staff constantly assesses the patient to ensure safety and an optimal setup for the particular surgery to be performed. To prevent inadvertent falls, the circulator applies a safety strap on the patient once the patient lies on the table. The circulator also regulates the room temperature and provides blankets for patient comfort and dignity. The scrub nurse sets up the back table, comprised of instruments and supplies needed for the procedure, while maintaining a sterile setup. The circulator is responsible for obtaining supplies requested by the anesthesia team, the surgeon, and the scrub tech, and also applies grounding pads to the patient for electrocautery equipment.

Surgeons and assistants often discuss particular nuances of the procedure to be performed at this time, as well as retrieve and display relevant imaging studies for the surgery. They should discuss positioning during the procedure and give an estimate of procedure length, indicating potential supply needs as well.

SECURING AND PADDING THE PATIENT TO THE TABLE

Ensuring that the patient is securely positioned on the table is of utmost importance. Falls from the OR table can have devastating consequences, resulting in injuries and long-term morbidity. Once the patient is anesthetized, she can no longer communicate pain or problems with positioning. The patient needs to be secured to the table with straps or bolsters, making sure to pad any pressure points. It is imperative that all team members aid in positioning and are comfortable with the final position of the patient.

Modern OR tables have built-in electric motors and can be moved in a variety of configurations. The table can be rolled side-to-side, positioned with the head or foot of the bed up, and even bent or flexed. As such, the team needs to test move the anesthetized patient into positions that are anticipated during the case before drapes are applied. This allows the team to verify secure patient placement on the table. Positioning for certain surgeries, such as those that require the patient to be placed in a lateral or Trendelenburg position (head down), carry a greater risk of falls from the OR table than those in which the patient is placed supine. The goal of positioning is to allow the best exposure for the surgeon while mitigating risk of falls, as well as compression and traction injuries, to the patient. Table 4.1 lists the most common surgical positions and their associated uses.

Supine Position

Supine positioning is one of the most common patient positions, used in a wide variety of surgeries. It creates adequate exposure for intra-abdominal surgeries, cardiothoracic procedures, some head and neck procedures, and procedures on the extremities. The patient is positioned lying face up (Fig. 4.1). From the supine

Table 4.1 Common Surgical Positions and Their Associated Uses

Patient Position	Procedures Utilizing Position
Supine	Majority of procedures, including chest, abdomen, and extremity surgeries
Prone	Percutaneous stone extraction; surgery of the back and spine
Trendelenburg	Robotic pelvic surgery, including prostatectomy and hysterectomy
Lateral	Procedures involving the hemithorax and retroperitoneum
Lithotomy	Transvaginal and transurethral procedures
Fowler's	Multiple ENT procedures; craniotomy; shoulder surgery

position, the table can be rotated laterally (side-to-side), placed in a slight Trendelenburg (head down) or reverse Trendelenburg (head up) position, or manipulated in various ways to gain exposure to the operative site. During pelvic procedures, for example, the table may be flexed or "broken" to gain better access and exposure to the pelvis (Fig. 4.2). A pillow is placed behind the knees to take tension off the thighs and lower back.

The patient's arms should be kept in a relaxed position on an arm board either perpendicular to the torso or at an angle toward the feet. Exposed arms give access to anesthesia for checking and placing lines and monitoring devices. Extending the arms to greater than 90 degrees creates the potential for brachial plexus injury and thus should be avoided. Tucking a patient's arms may be necessary if they inhibit access of the surgical team to the operative field or when using equipment such as a C-arm fluoroscopy unit. Although rare, this exposes the hands to pinching injuries from bed components and compartment syndrome if placed under the buttocks.

Prone Position

The prone position is common for use in surgeries that involve the back and spine. The patient is positioned such that the abdomen and chest are facing downward on the OR table (Fig. 4.3). Induction and reversal of anesthesia are usually accomplished with the patient in the supine position on the OR table or another table from which the patient will then be flipped onto the OR table and into the prone position. From the prone position, the patient can be placed in a jackknife position for cases that involve access to the anus and rectum (Fig. 4.4).

Taking care to prevent complications from prone positioning is extremely important, especially when a lengthy procedure is expected. Recognized complications include perioperative visual loss, brachial plexus nerve injury, and ulnar nerve injury. Albeit rare, less

common injuries include myocutaneous complications such as pressure ulcers and compartment syndrome.[1] Most of these complications are easily preventable, however, with strict attention to detail while padding pressure points and ensuring that little traction is placed on the extremities. In women, it is important to properly pad the breasts and ensure that the nipples are moved laterally to avoid pressure necrosis. In addition, chest rolls placed parallel to the torso from each shoulder to the waist can help provide space for chest and lung expansion during prolonged procedures (Fig. 4.5).

Trendelenburg Position

Named after the German surgeon Friedrich Trendelenburg, who first described the position, the Trendelenburg position is a modification of the supine position.[2] The patient is first placed supine, then after securely fastening the patient in place to the OR table, the head of the bed is tilted 15 to 30 degrees downward (Fig. 4.6). This allows abdominal viscera to displace cephalad and aids in lower abdominal and pelvic procedures, such as abdominal hysterectomy and prostate procedures. The patient's legs may be kept on the OR table or placed in stirrups to allow perineal exposure and provide additional support from sliding cephalad on the table.

Considerations for positioning in the Trendelenburg position include increased central venous return, increased intracranial pressure, increased intraocular pressure, increased pulmonary venous pressure and decreased pulmonary compliance, and increased myocardial work.[3–7] The likelihood of complications arising from Trendelenburg positioning increases with longer procedures, as well as steeper positioning.

Conversely, reverse Trendelenburg displaces abdominal viscera caudally. This can aid in exposure of upper abdominal contents, such as is required in gastric surgery. This position causes pooling of blood in the lower extremities and creates an increased risk of deep venous thrombosis (DVT).[8] It is therefore imperative that compression stockings be used in procedures that involve the reverse Trendelenburg position.

Lateral Position

The lateral position provides exposure to the hemithorax and retroperitoneal structures such as the kidneys and ureters. Positioning involves first intubating the patient while supine, then turning the patient to the correct side. The dependent side conveys the name of the procedure such that patients positioned with the right side down are in the right lateral decubitus position, whereas patients positioned with the left side down are in the left lateral decubitus position (Fig. 4.7).

It is especially important when positioning a patient into the lateral decubitus position to securely

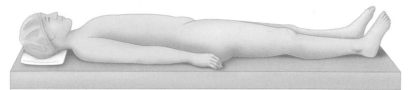

Fig. 4.1 Supine position

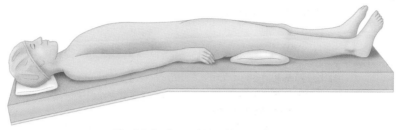

Fig. 4.2 Supine position with table flexed

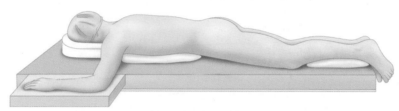

Fig. 4.3 Prone position

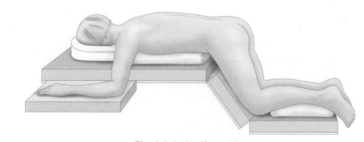

Fig. 4.4 Jackknife position

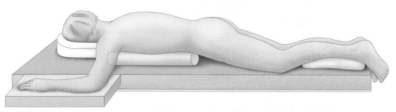

Fig. 4.5 Chest rolls used to support the torso and provide room for chest and lung expansion

fasten the patient to the OR table while minimizing traction and pressure to various areas. Tape may be used for this purpose, as it allows for flexibility in patient body habitus while having enough strength to ensure that the patient does not move once fastened to the table. Numerous different areas should be used to fasten the patient to the table, including at the legs, hips, and chest. A towel should be placed between the skin and tape to avoid skin trauma, as with prolonged tension and swelling skin disruption and burns can occur. It is important to maintain the patient's head in a neutral position to the rest of the body and preserve cervical spine and body alignment. This can be accomplished via use of a combination of pillows, blankets, and foam and gel donuts.

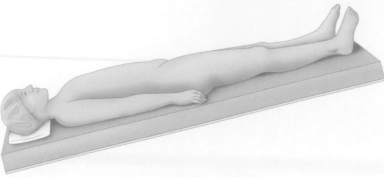

Fig. 4.6 Trendelenburg position

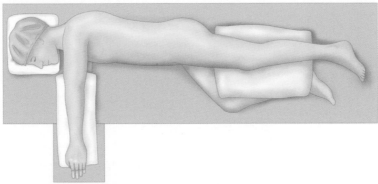

Fig. 4.7 Patient positioned in the full lateral decubitus position

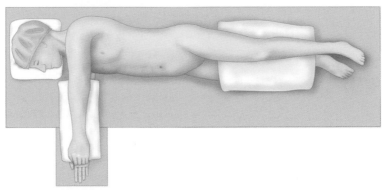

Fig. 4.8 Patient positioned in the modified lateral decubitus position

To support the patient's torso and back, a gel roll may be placed between the patient's back and the OR table. The legs should be positioned so that the lower leg is slightly bent at the knee while the upper leg is maintained in extension. During surgeries that involve positioning in a modified flank position so that the patient is lateralized on the table but not completely on his side, the legs may both be left extended on the OR table with a pillow used for support at the knees (Fig. 4.8).

Positioning of the arms is also important, as injuries to the brachial plexus can occur. The lower arm is usually placed outstretched on an arm board,

perpendicular to the torso. It can be padded, particularly at the elbow, with convoluted (egg crate) foam material to minimize pressure. The upper extremity should be relaxed with the palm facing downward and may be supported in a variety of ways. In the full lateral position, blankets placed between the arms may be used (Fig. 4.9). Alternatively, an elevated support such as an arm rest may be utilized (Fig. 4.10). In patients positioned in the modified flank position, oftentimes the arm may be rested on the torso for support and may be secured in a sling made of a towel and tape (Fig. 4.11).

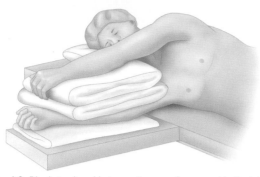

Fig. 4.9 Blankets placed between the arms for support in the lateral decubitus position

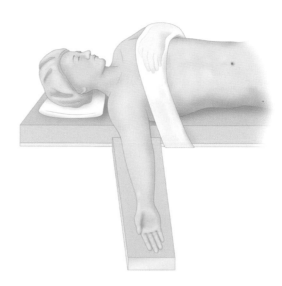

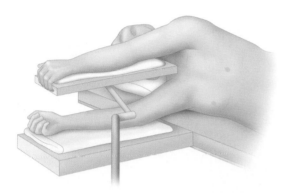

Fig. 4.10 Arm rest used for support in the lateral decubitus position

Fig. 4.11 Sling made of a towel and tape for arm support

Lithotomy Position

The dorsal lithotomy position provides excellent exposure for perineal, perirectal/anal, transvaginal, and transurethral procedures. After inducing anesthesia in the supine position, the patient's knees are flexed, and the hips are flexed and slightly abducted while being elevated to provide exposure (Fig. 4.12). Various types of lithotomy stirrups can be used, including those that provide support for the entire leg (Fig. 4.13), only the knee, or straps that suspend the legs by the feet (see Fig. 4.12). It is important to minimize pressure on the lateral knee, posterior leg, and ankle while in the lithotomy position. Compression of the lateral knee can lead to injury of the common peroneal nerve, resulting in foot drop. Factors associated with this include a larger body habitus and longer duration in the lithotomy position.[9] It is also important to avoid hyperabduction of the hips.

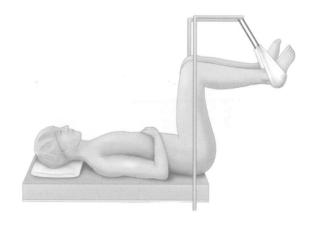

Fig. 4.12 Lithotomy position

Fowler's Position

Fowler's position, or the seated position, is used for certain shoulder, head and neck, and cranial neurosurgical procedures. It allows optimal access to these sites while promoting drainage from the surgical site. After anesthesia is induced in the supine position, the patient is secured to the table and then positioned as if in a chair

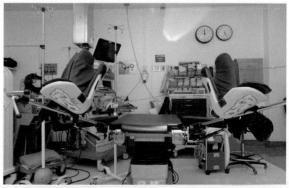

Fig. 4.13 Leg supports for use in the lithotomy position

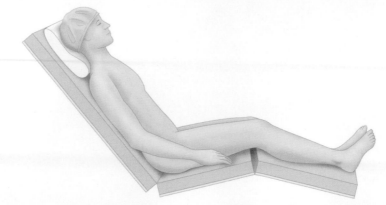

Fig. 4.14 Fowler's position

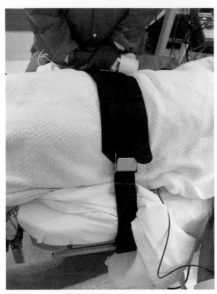

Fig. 4.15 Table strap

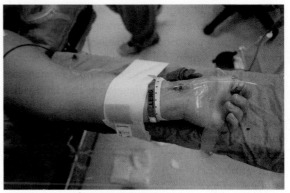

Fig. 4.16 Arm straps

(Fig. 4.14). Complications are usually rare but may include pressure ulcers during prolonged surgeries and, in very rare cases, venous air embolism.[10]

General Considerations

Regardless of the position in which the patient is to be placed, it is imperative to securely fasten the patient to the table to prevent slips and falls during the procedure. Additionally, during reversal of anesthesia, it is not uncommon for a patient to begin to move on the OR table. It is for this reason that patients need to be secured to the table and monitored at all times by OR personnel. Various materials can be used for securing the patient to the table, including surgical table straps, arm straps, and tape. Surgical table straps can be reusable or single use, and can be made of nylon, vinyl, cloth, or other materials (Fig. 4.15). Certain positions dictate that the patient should be more securely fastened to the OR table, including the lateral, Trendelenburg, and Fowler's positions. Silk or cloth tape, as well as

other strong adhesives, can be used for this purpose. During procedures in which the arms are to be maintained on arm boards, arm straps should be used to prevent the arms from falling, which could result in injuries or contamination of the sterile field (Fig. 4.16).

During positioning, pressure should be minimized to prevent skin ulceration. Whereas the supine position distributes weight more evenly across the entire back and lower extremities, positions such as lateral decubitus and prone distribute pressure less evenly and across bony prominences, where injuries are more likely to occur. Padding of areas such as the breasts in females and the genitalia in males during prone procedures is recommended to reduce such injuries. Preventing pressure injuries can be accomplished via use of corrugated foam pads; pillows and blankets; and gel rolls, pads, and donuts (Fig. 4.17). Padding the heels to prevent ulcers should also be performed and can be achieved by placing heel pads on the patient at the outset of the procedure (Fig. 4.18).

ANESTHESIA LINES AND TUBES

The anesthesia team serves a critical role in the OR. Tasked with airway management, vascular access, patient monitoring, and inducing a state of analgesia,

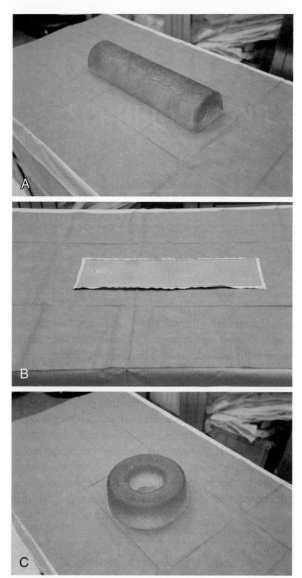

Fig. 4.17 Gel supports used to reduce pressure injuries. A. Gel roll. B. Gel pad. C. Gel donut.

amnesia, paralysis, and unconsciousness, surgery would not be possible without anesthesia. Common vascular access, airway management, and patient monitoring devices are discussed here.

Vascular Access

IV access allows fluids to be administered to maintain patient hydration, as well as to administer medications for sedation, induction of anesthesia, amnesia, paralysis, and pain/nausea control. IV access can be started in the preoperative holding area or after the patient enters the OR. IV cannulas are available in a variety of sizes, ranging commonly from 14 to 24 gauge (G). By convention, larger cannulas are numbered in decreasing order, such that a 14G angiocatheter is larger than a 20G angiocatheter (Fig. 4.19).

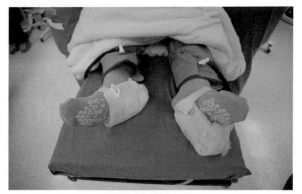

Fig. 4.18 Heel pads

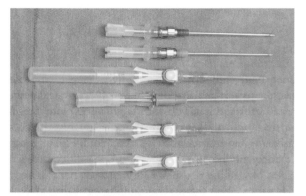

Fig. 4.19 IV cannulas

During routine cases in which minimal blood loss is expected, one peripheral IV line, typically placed in the arm, is usually adequate. When venous access is limited, lines may be placed in the foot or leg. Although larger access is always preferred in case of emergency, an 18 or 20G IV is usually sufficient for most procedures. During more involved, complex cases with the potential for a greater blood loss, at least two large-bore (18G or larger) IVs should be placed. Trauma cases that require delivering a large amount of IV fluids and blood products over a short period of time necessitate as large an IV as possible, usually with two or more sites of access.

Central venous catheters, also known as central lines, are available for placement in patients with numerous comorbidities and/or those undergoing complex surgeries. They allow the delivery of large amounts of IV fluids, blood products, and medications over a short period of time. Additionally, they allow, when needed, for a steady delivery of medication via a pump, such as vasopressors (medications to increase BP). In the OR, central lines are usually placed in the internal jugular or subclavian veins, although they may also be placed in the femoral vein. Ultrasound guidance is often used to facilitate placement. Central lines typically range in size between 14G and 22G, and may have one, two, or three ports. They should not be confused with a peripheral

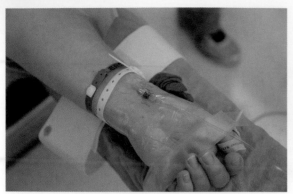

Fig. 4.20 Radial artery arterial line

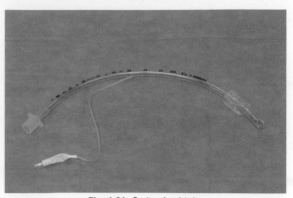

Fig. 4.21 Orotracheal tube

external jugular vein IV, which can look similar to a central line but has the limitations of a peripheral line.

Arterial lines (also known as A-lines or art-lines) are used to monitor BP in real time and for obtaining samples for arterial blood gas (ABG) analysis. They are commonly placed in the radial artery at the wrist (Fig. 4.20) but can also be placed in the ulnar artery, brachial artery, or femoral artery if necessary. They are used to facilitate monitoring when fluctuations in BP may occur, such as in procedures with high estimated blood loss or in individuals with medical issues that can affect BP. Medications and fluids, however, cannot be administered through arterial lines.

Airway Management

There are various methods of managing the airway during surgery. If there is epidural or spinal anesthesia, oxygen via a nasal cannula or mask may be sufficient. For a general anesthetic, the mainstay of airway management has long been endotracheal intubation with an endotracheal (ET) tube. With proper airway access, anesthetics and other medications can be administered into the lungs. The patient can be ventilated either by mechanical ventilation or by hand, and the airway is protected from aspiration and asphyxiation. The most commonly used route is via orotracheal intubation with a tube passed through the oropharynx (Fig. 4.21). Nasotracheal intubation can also be used in patients undergoing procedures necessitating access to the mouth or in patients with conditions that prevent orotracheal intubation, such as laryngeal cancer or stenosis. In patients with a previously placed tracheostomy, ventilation and the delivery of medications can be accomplished through the tracheostomy directly.

In some cases where definitive control of the airway is not necessary and the duration of the procedure is expected to be short, the decision to provide bag-mask ventilation may be appropriate. Instead of placing an

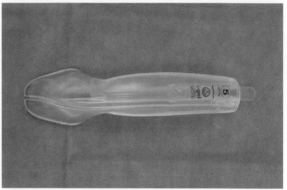

Fig. 4.22 Laryngeal mask airway

ET tube or laryngeal mask airway (LMA), a mask is placed over the nose and mouth, and the anesthesia provider ventilates the patient via a bag. Advantages to this method include minimal trauma and quick airway management. Disadvantages, however, are related primarily to the limited control of the airway provided by bag-mask ventilation, gastric distention from pressurized ventilation, and provider fatigue if the procedure is lengthy.

The LMA device (Fig. 4.22) is an alternative to bag-mask ventilation in which better control of the airway is achieved but does not necessitate complete endotracheal intubation. An LMA is a supraglottic device that sits in the hypopharynx, allowing relative isolation of the trachea for ventilation. Less gastric distention occurs than with bag-mask ventilation, and the anesthesia provider does not need to actively ventilate the patient. Relative contraindications to LMA ventilation are prolonged procedures where the risk of aspiration is greater, morbid obesity, and in patients who have not fasted prior to anesthesia induction.[11]

Patient Monitoring

Along with providing anesthesia during a surgical procedure, the anesthesia team serves a critical role in

Table 4.2 Vital Signs Monitored During Surgery

Vital Sign	Normal Range	How It Is Measured	Notes
Temperature	36.1–37.9°C	Axillary, oral, rectal, or skin thermometer	Should be checked sporadically during surgical case
Blood pressure	90–140/60–90	Blood pressure cuff; arterial line	Continuously monitored with arterial line; sporadically monitored with blood pressure cuff
Heart rate	60–100 beats/min	Pulse oximeter; telemetry, arterial line	Continuously monitored
Respiratory rate	12–20 breaths/min	Ventilator	May be controlled by the anesthesia provider through the ventilator
Oxygen saturation	95–100%	Pulse oximeter	Continuously monitored
Heart rhythm		Telemetry; EKG	Visually monitored for arrhythmias

monitoring the patient's vital signs. Anesthesia providers monitor several different patient parameters during a surgical procedure, including BP, heart rate (HR) and rhythm, oxygen saturation, and ABG values. Table 4.2 shows the vital signs monitored during a surgery, including how they are measured. It is imperative that the surgeon and anesthesia provider communicate effectively throughout a procedure to ensure optimal patient outcomes. If a surgeon expects a particular part of a procedure to involve a greater blood loss than other parts of the procedure, communication to the anesthesia provider allows preparation for additional fluids or blood products and necessary medications to support pressure. By the same token, the anesthesia provider should effectively and immediately communicate with the surgeon any change in the patient's status during the procedure to mitigate any potential risks to the patient.

Typically, BP is measured during the course of an operation via a BP cuff placed on the arm or leg. Ensuring an appropriately sized cuff allows accurate BP monitoring. BP cuffs that are too large risk reporting BP measurements that are lower than the true BP, whereas cuffs that are too small risk reporting higher BP measurements than the true BP. BP cuffs cycle throughout the course of an operation and do not provide continuous real-time BP monitoring.

Alternatively, arterial lines provide a continuous real-time view of a patient's BP throughout the course of a procedure. Whereas BP cuffs are used in nearly every procedure, arterial lines are placed for procedures that require closer BP monitoring. In contrast to BP cuffs, arterial lines also measure a patient's HR.

Pulse oximetry is a reliable way to measure arterial oxygen saturation (O_2 sat) and HR. Oximeters are usually placed on the fingers, although sometimes they are placed on the earlobe or forehead. They provide information in real time and are quick and easy to place.

Cardiac monitoring (telemetry) requires the placement of three or more leads on the chest and extremities (Fig. 4.23). Cardiac monitoring occurs in real time

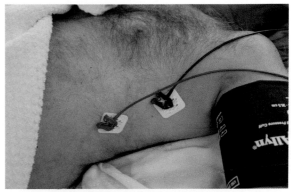

Fig. 4.23 Two telemetry leads placed on a patient for cardiac monitoring during surgery

and monitors both HR and rhythm. Abnormalities can signal significant cardiovascular compromise, including significant intravascular depletion from blood loss, arrhythmias, or myocardial injury.

ABG monitoring is common during surgeries that involve prolonged anesthesia times, thoracic procedures, and the potential for significant blood loss. In cases where ABG monitoring is expected, an arterial line is usually placed for ease of obtaining a sample. Important information obtained from ABG testing includes pH, arterial oxygen partial pressure (P_aO_2), arterial carbon dioxide partial pressure (P_aCO_2), and bicarbonate (HCO_3^-) content. Additional tests can be requested, as needed, including lactate, hemoglobin and hematocrit, and electrolyte levels. Table 4.3 provides a comprehensive review of ABG parameters commonly assessed during surgery.

DVT PREVENTION

The development of a DVT in the perioperative period is a significant cause of morbidity and mortality. Pulmonary embolism (PE) as a result of DVT remains the most commonly preventable cause of hospital death.[12–14] Numerous risk factors for DVT exist in surgical patients, including prolonged immobility both during and after surgery, advanced age, vascular insult creating a hypercoagulable state, malignancy, pregnancy, a history of DVT, and inherited or acquired hypercoagulable states.[15–19] Recent American College of Chest Physicians (ACCP) guidelines define surgical patients as either very low risk, low risk, moderate risk, or high risk for developing a DVT following surgery. The modified Caprini risk assessment model (Table 4.4) defines several risk factors for developing a DVT and assigns each a numeric score. The total score represents a patient's overall risk of developing a DVT and places a patient in a particular risk category. Very low risk patients are those with a Caprini score of 0 and have an estimated 0.5% risk of developing a DVT. Low risk patients are those with a Caprini score of 1 to 2 and have an estimated 1.5% risk of developing a DVT. Moderate risk is defined as a Caprini score of 3 to 4 and carries approximately 3% risk of developing a DVT. High risk is defined as a Caprini score ≥5 and represents approximately 6% risk of developing a DVT.[20]

Prophylaxis against venous thromboembolism (VTE) can be characterized as either mechanical or pharmacologic. The easiest mechanical means is early ambulation. Additional mechanical methods of prophylaxis include intermittent pneumatic compression (IPC) devices, compression stockings, and the venous foot pump. Any of these can be used in combination with pharmacologic prophylaxis when necessary. IPC should be started in the OR prior to induction of anesthesia and usually continues through the hospital stay (Fig. 4.24). Mechanical compressive prophylaxis is contraindicated, however, in patients with a current DVT.

Table 4.3 ABG Parameters Assessed During Surgery

Parameter	Normal Range
pH	7.34–7.44
H+	35–45 nmol/L
Arterial partial pressure of oxygen (P_aO_2)	75–100 mm Hg
Arterial partial pressure of carbon dioxide (P_aCO_2)	35–45 mm Hg
Bicarbonate (HCO_3-)	22–26 mEq/L
Base excess	–2 to +2 mmol/L
Hemoglobin	12.0–17.5 g/dL
Hematocrit	35–50%
Lactate	0.5–1.0 mmol/L
Sodium	135–145 mEq/L
Potassium	3.5–5.0 mEq/L
Chloride	97–107
Glucose	70–99

Table 4.4 Modified Caprini Risk Assessment Model

Caprini risk assessment model

1 Point	2 Points	3 Points	5 Points
Age 41–60 years	Age 61–74 years	Age ≥75 years	Stroke (<1 month)
Minor surgery	Arthroscopic surgery	History of venous thromboembolism	Elective arthroplasty
Body mass index >25 kg/m^2	Major open surgery (>45 min)	Family history of venous thromboembolism	Hip, pelvis, or leg fracture
Swollen legs	Laparoscopic surgery (>45 min)	Factor V Leiden	Acute spinal cord injury (<1 month)
Varicose veins	Malignancy	Prothrombin 2021 0A	
Pregnancy or postpartum	Confined to bed (>72 h)	Lupus anticoagulant	
History of unexplained or recurrent spontaneous abortion	Immobilizing plaster cast	Anticardiolipin antibodies	
Oral contraceptives or hormone replacement	Central venous access	Elevated serum homocysteine	
Sepsis (<1 month)		Heparin-induced thrombocytopenia	
Serious lung disease, including pneumonia (<1 month)		Other congenital or acquired thrombophilia	
Abnormal pulmonary function			
Acute myocardial infarction			
Congestive heart failure (<1 month)			
History of inflammatory bowel disease			
Medical patient at bed rest			

Reproduced with permission from Gould MK, Garcia DA, Wren SM, et al. Prevention of VTE in nonorthopedic surgical patients: Antithrombotic Therapy and Prevention of Thrombosis, 9th ed: American College of Chest Physicians Evidence-Based Clinical Practice Guidelines. Chest. 2012;141(suppl 2):e227S–e277S.

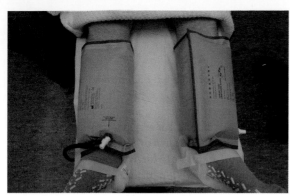

Fig. 4.24 IPC device

Pharmacologic prophylaxis against VTE includes unfractionated subcutaneous heparin, low-molecular-weight heparin, fondaparinux, warfarin, and other vitamin K antagonists.[20] In general, in patients considered to be at very low risk for the development of a DVT, ACCP guidelines recommend that no postoperative prophylaxis against VTE be used outside of early ambulation. In patients at low risk, ACCP guidelines recommend mechanical prophylaxis alone over no prophylaxis at all. In patients at moderate risk and in whom the risk of severe bleeding complications is low, ACCP guidelines recommend pharmacologic prophylaxis over mechanical prophylaxis. In patients at moderate risk and in whom the risk of bleeding is high, mechanical prophylaxis should be used until the risk of bleeding is acceptable, at which time pharmacologic prophylaxis should be started. In patients at high risk for VTE and in whom the risk of major bleeding is low, pharmacologic prophylaxis in combination with mechanical prophylaxis should be used. In patients at high risk and in whom the risk of bleeding is high, mechanical prophylaxis should be used until the risk of bleeding is acceptable, at which time pharmacologic prophylaxis should be started.

In patients with a high risk of bleeding complications following surgery and in whom the risk of developing a DVT is high, consideration should be given to preoperative placement of an inferior vena cava (IVC) filter. This is particularly applicable in patients with a current DVT or with a history of DVT. IVC filters can be either permanent or retrievable, allowing them to be removed after surgery.

ANTIBIOTICS

Surgical site infections (SSIs) can be the cause of significant morbidity after a procedure. At the same time, the emergence of resistant organisms and antibiotic-associated infections such as *Clostridium difficile* colitis cautions against the widespread general use of antibiotics. It is the role of practitioners to determine the optimal type and duration of antibiotic prophylaxis for each surgical procedure. Although certain procedures may not require antibiotic prophylaxis at all, some may require coverage with multiple agents directed against typical flora at the surgical site.

Most surgical procedures can be classified into one of four general wound classifications: clean, clean-contaminated, contaminated, or dirty. Clean procedures involve an uninfected space in which the wound is closed primarily. An example of a clean procedure is an excision of a skin lesion and carries a 1.3 to 2.9% rate of wound infection. Clean-contaminated procedures are those that involve controlled entry into either the respiratory, gastrointestinal (GI), or genitourinary tract. There is no unusual contamination during these procedures. Examples of clean-contaminated surgeries include gastric surgery, colon surgery, bronchoscopy, and cystoscopy. There is a 2.4 to 7.7% risk of wound infection with a clean-contaminated wound. Contaminated procedures are those that incur a major break in sterile technique; involve gross spillage from the GI tract; or involve an open, fresh, accidental wound. Examples of contaminated surgeries include appendectomy for acute appendicitis, spillage of bile during a cholecystectomy, and penetrating wounds. There is a 6.4 to 15.2% risk of wound infection with a contaminated wound. Dirty procedures are those that involve an existing infection, a perforated viscus, fecal contamination, retained devitalized tissue from a previous wound, or foreign bodies. These include surgeries in which there is a perforated bowel with gross spillage of contents, abscess incision and drainage, wound debridement, and in cases where there is a positive preoperative culture of the surgical site. Dirty wounds carry a 7.1 to 40.0% risk of wound infection.[21–24]

The choice of antibiotic for a surgical procedure should be based on the typical organisms residing at the surgical site. Skin flora, such as coagulase-negative staphylococci, *Staphylococcus aureus*, and streptococcal species, are the most common cause of SSI.[25] Choosing an antibiotic with activity against these organisms is therefore important. First-generation cephalosporins, such as cefazolin, are widely used for procedural antibiotic prophylaxis because they have good coverage against most bacteria, have a favorable and long duration of action, and are cost effective. Most antibiotics should be administered within 60 minutes of incision to optimize tissue levels, although certain antibiotics such as vancomycin require a longer infusion time and should be initiated sooner. Additionally, repeat dosing of some antibiotics should occur if the half-life of the antibiotic is short and the surgery is sufficiently long. Postoperatively, most patients should not receive further antibiotic prophylaxis, although continued antibiotic prophylaxis might be warranted in patients undergoing dirty, contaminated, and certain clean-contaminated procedures.

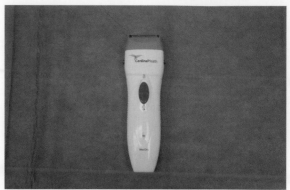

Fig. 4.25 Clippers for preoperative hair removal

SKIN SHAVING

Hair removal is considered an important part of preoperative preparation in those areas in which hair would interfere with the surgical incision, skin closure, and procedure itself. For this reason, it is important to remove hair in these areas just prior to incision, as SSI is reduced when hair is removed immediately preceding incision as compared to in advance.[26] Additionally, the method of hair removal has been shown to be important in reducing SSI. As compared to skin shaving with a razor, which causes greater trauma to skin surfaces, hair removal with clippers has been shown to decrease the rate of SSI.[27] Thus, in cases in which hair removal is necessary, clippers are preferred (Fig. 4.25).

SKIN STERILIZATION

An additional part of the immediate preoperative preparation includes surgical site skin disinfection. After hair removal, skin sterilization can be performed with either a chlorhexidine-containing solution or an iodine-based solution. Several recent studies have compared the rate of SSI after skin sterilization with either chlorhexidine or iodine, and have found that the use of chlorhexidine-containing solutions results in a lower incidence of SSI (relative risk of ~0.6) compared to iodine-containing solutions.[28-30] For this reason, it is typically recommended that chlorhexidine be used for preoperative skin decontamination when possible. An exception to this is when disinfection of a mucous membrane is required. In this case, chlorhexidine has resulted in increased rates of allergic reactions, and the use of iodine-containing solutions is preferred.[31,32] All loose hair and debris should be removed from the operative field. The area should be prepared widely in the unanticipated event that an incision needs to be made longer. Painting with a solution needs to start at the center of the operative field and be covered by making concentric circles (see Chapter 3). It is important to give adequate time for the agent to dry.

THE TIME OUT

The surgical time out is an integral part of ensuring patient safety prior to the start of a procedure. It is only in extremely urgent and rare situations that the time out may be omitted, such as in cases when life or limb is imminently threatened. Prior to the start of all elective and most emergency surgeries, the time out serves at minimum to reidentify the patient, surgical team, proposed surgery, site of surgery, and laterality of the procedure, if present. It also acts to ensure that important safety measures have been implemented, such as the administration of antibiotics and antithrombosis prophylaxis. Surgical time outs have been shown to prevent wrong-side surgeries, improve communication between team members, and even increase patient satisfaction.[33]

During the time-out process, no other activities should be occurring and individuals are discouraged from entering or leaving the room. The time out usually takes place once the surgical team is scrubbed, the patient is prepped and draped for surgery, and equipment is set up, but prior to an incision being made. All team members identify themselves, and a checklist is reviewed (Fig. 4.26). If the procedure includes multiple steps, and especially when the patient is repositioned on the OR table, a second time out, or modified "mini" time out, may be performed to reconfirm the procedure and laterality. Additionally, numerous institutions have begun to implement a sign-out process at the conclusion of surgery that reconfirms the correct procedure, laterality, implants if used, specimens, and estimated blood loss, and documents any complications and the remedies used to mitigate them.

Surgical safety checklist

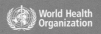 **World Health Organization** | **Patient Safety**
A World Alliance for Safer Health Care

Before induction of anaesthesia	Before skin incision	Before patient leaves operating room
(with at least nurse and anaesthetist)	(with nurse, anaesthetist and surgeon)	(with nurse, anaesthetist and surgeon)

Before induction of anaesthesia

Has the patient confirmed his/her identity, site, procedure, and consent?
☐ Yes

Is the site marked?
☐ Yes
☐ Not applicable

Is the anaesthesia machine and medication check complete?
☐ Yes

Is the pulse oximeter on the patient and functioning?
☐ Yes

Does the patient have a:

Known allergy?
☐ No
☐ Yes

Difficult airway or aspiration risk?
☐ No
☐ Yes, and equipment/assistance available

Risk of >500ml blood loss (7ml/kg in children)?
☐ No
☐ Yes, and two IVs/central access and fluids planned

Before skin incision

☐ Confirm all team members have introduced themselves by name and role.
☐ Confirm the patient's name, procedure, and where the incision will be made.

Has antibiotic prophylaxis been given within the last 60 minutes?
☐ Yes
☐ Not applicable

Anticipated critical events

To surgeon:
☐ What are the critical or non-routine steps?
☐ How long will the case take?
☐ What is the anticipated blood loss?

To anaesthetist:
☐ Are there any patient-specific concerns?

To nursing team:
☐ Has sterility (including indicator results) been confirmed?
☐ Are there equipment issues or any concerns?

Is essential imaging displayed?
☐ Yes
☐ Not applicable

Before patient leaves operating room

Nurse verbally confirms:
☐ The name of the procedure
☐ Completion of instrument, sponge and needle counts
☐ Specimen labelling (read specimen labels aloud, including patient name)
☐ Whether there are any equipment problems to be addressed

To surgeon, anaesthetist and nurse:
☐ What are the key concerns for recovery and management of this patient?

This checklist is not intended to be comprehensive. Additions and modifications to fit local practice are encouraged. Revised 1 / 2009 © WHO, 2009

Fig. 4.26 Surgical time-out checklist. Reproduced with permission from http://www.who.int/patientsafety/safesurgery/checklist/en/

REFERENCES

1. DePasse JM, Palumbo MA, Haque M, Eberson CP, Daniels AH. Complications associated with prone positioning in elective spinal surgery. *World Journal of Orthopedics.* 2015;6(3):351–359.
2. Friedrich Trendelenburg (1844–1924). Trendelenburg's position. *Journal of the American Medical Association.* 1969;207(6):1143–1144.
3. Awad H, Santilli S, Ohr M, et al. The effects of steep Trendelenburg positioning on intraocular pressure during robotic radical prostatectomy. *Anesthesia and Analgesia.* 2009;109(2):473–478.
4. Choi SJ, Gwak MS, Ko JS, et al. The effects of the exaggerated lithotomy position for radical perineal prostatectomy on respiratory mechanics. *Anaesthesia.* 2006;61(5):439–443.
5. Kalmar AF, Foubert L, Hendrickx JF, et al. Influence of steep Trendelenburg position and CO(2) pneumoperitoneum on cardiovascular, cerebrovascular, and respiratory homeostasis during robotic prostatectomy. *British Journal of Anaesthesia.* 2010;104(4):433–439.
6. Kaye AD, Anesthetic considerations in robotic-assisted gynecologic surgery. *Ochner Journal.* 2013;13(4):517–524.
7. Molloy BL. Implications for postoperative visual loss: steep Trendelenburg position and effects on intraocular pressure. *AANA Journal.* 2011;79(2):115–121.
8. Catheline JM, Capelluto E, Gaillard JL, Turner R, Champault G. Thromboembolism prophylaxis and incidence of thromboembolic complications after laparoscopic surgery. *International Journal of Surgical Investigation.* 2000;2(1):41–47.
9. Warner MA, Martin JT, Schroeder DR, Offord KP, Chute CG. Lower-extremity motor neuropathy associated with surgery performed on patients in a lithotomy position. *Anesthesiology.* 1994;81(1):6–12.
10. Ammirati M, Lamki TT, Shaw AB, Forde B, Nakano I, Mani M. A streamlined protocol for the use of the semi-sitting position in neurosurgery: a report on 48 consecutive procedures. *Journal of Clinical Neuroscience.* 2013;20(1):32–34.
11. Pollack Jr CV. The laryngeal mask airway: a comprehensive review for the emergency physician. *Journal of Emergency Medicine.* 2001;20(1):53–66.
12. Lindblad B, Eriksson A, Bergqvist D. Autopsy-verified pulmonary embolism in a surgical department: analysis of the period from 1951 to 1988. *British Journal of Surgery.* 1991;78(7):849–852.
13. Martino MA, Borges E, Williamson E, et al. Pulmonary embolism after major abdominal surgery in gynecologic oncology. *Obstetrics and Gynecology.* 2006;107(3):666–671.
14. Sandler DA, Martin JF. Autopsy proven pulmonary embolism in hospital patients: are we detecting enough deep vein thrombosis? *Journal of the Royal Society of Medicine.* 1989;82(4):203–205.
15. Anderson Jr FA, Spencer FA. Risk factors for venous thromboembolism. *Circulation.* 2003;107(23 suppl 1):I9–I16.
16. Cook D, Crowther M, Meade M, et al. Deep venous thrombosis in medical-surgical critically ill patients: prevalence, incidence, and risk factors. *Critical Care Medicine.* 2005;33(7):1565–1571.
17. McColl MD, Walker ID, Greer IA. Risk factors for venous thromboembolism in pregnancy. *Current Opinion in Pulmonary Medicine.* 1999;5(4):227–232.
18. Osborne NH, Wakefield TW, Henke PK. Venous thromboembolism in cancer patients undergoing major surgery. *Annals of Surgical Oncology.* 2008;15(12):3567–3578.
19. Petralia GA, Kakkar AK. Venous thromboembolism prophylaxis for the general surgical patient: where do we stand? *Seminars in Respiratory and Critical Care Medicine.* 2008;29(1):83–89.

20. Gould MK, Garcia DA, Wren SM, et al. Prevention of VTE in nonorthopedic surgical patients: Antithrombotic Therapy and Prevention of Thrombosis, 9th ed. American College of Chest Physicians Evidence-Based Clinical Practice Guidelines. *Chest.* 2012;141(suppl 2):e227S–e277S.

21. Cruse PJ, Foord R. The epidemiology of wound infection. A 10-year prospective study of 62,939 wounds. *Surgical Clinics of North America.* 1980;60(1):27–40.

22. Culver DH, Horan TC, Gaynes RP, et al. Surgical wound infection rates by wound class, operative procedure, and patient risk index. National Nosocomial Infections Surveillance System. *American Journal of Medicine.* 1991;91(3b):152s–157s.

23. Haley RW, Culver DH, Morgan WM, White JW, Emori TG, Hooton TM. Identifying patients at high risk of surgical wound infection. A simple multivariate index of patient susceptibility and wound contamination. *American Journal of Epidemiology.* 1985;121(2):206–215.

24. Olson M, O'Connor M, Schwartz ML. Surgical wound infections. A 5-year prospective study of 20,193 wounds at the Minneapolis VA Medical Center. *Annals of Surgery.* 1984;199(3):253–259.

25. Hidron AI, Edwards JR, Patel J, et al. NHSN annual update: antimicrobial-resistant pathogens associated with healthcare-associated infections. Annual summary of data reported to the National Healthcare Safety Network at the Centers for Disease Control and Prevention, 2006–2007. *Infection Control and Hospital Epidemiology.* 2008;29(11):996–1011.

26. Seropian R, Reynolds BM. Wound infections after preoperative depilatory versus razor preparation. *American Journal of Surgery.* 1971;121(3):251–254.

27. Tanner J, Woodings D, Moncaster K. Preoperative hair removal to reduce surgical site infection. *Cochrane Database of Systematic Reviews.* 2006;(3):CD004122.

28. Darouiche RO, Wall Jr MJ, Itani KM, et al. Chlorhexidine-alcohol versus povidone-iodine for surgical-site antisepsis. *New England Journal of Medicine.* 2010;362(1):18–26.

29. Noorani A, Rabey N, Walsh SR, Davies RJ. Systematic review and meta-analysis of preoperative antisepsis with chlorhexidine versus povidone-iodine in clean-contaminated surgery. *British Journal of Surgery.* 2010;97(11):1614–1620.

30. Srinivas A, Kaman L, Raj P, et al. Comparison of the efficacy of chlorhexidine gluconate versus povidone iodine as preoperative skin preparation for the prevention of surgical site infections in clean-contaminated upper abdominal surgeries. *Surgery Today.* 2015;45(11):1378–1384.

31. Rutkowski K, Wagner A. Chlorhexidine: a new latex? *European Urology.* 2015;68(3):345–347.

32. Wicki J, Deluze C, Cirafici L, Desmeules J. Anaphylactic shock induced by intraurethral use of chlorhexidine. *Allergy.* 1999;54(7):768–769.

33. Kozusko SD, Elkwood L, Gaynor D, Chagares SA. An innovative approach to the surgical time out: a patient-focused model. *AORN Journal.* 2016;103(6):617–622.

CHAPTER 5

BASIC TOOLS OF THE TRADE AND HOW TO USE THEM

Surgical instruments have evolved to permit precise surgery under direct vision. These instruments allow dissection and reconstruction beyond the capability of bare human hands. They can allow the surgeon to modulate force placed on tissue, see in deep incisions by virtue of their narrow profile, and keep hands away from tissue to minimize the risk of contamination of both the surgical wound and healthcare personnel.

Surgical instruments are meticulously crafted and precision engineered. As with any tool, learning proper technique for use, as well as practice, is necessary for mastery. One must also become familiar with the specific purpose for each instrument. In general, instruments fall into defined categories that, when used in concert, allow for successful and safe surgery. Through the evolution of surgery, the same instrument may be called by a different name in different regions of the country or world. For example, the mosquito clamp is often referred to as a Crile, Pean, Rochester, stat, or snap depending on surgeon and hospital preference. Video 5.1 demonstrates the proper manner in which to hold various surgical instruments.

Surgical hand tools are constructed of stainless steel to resist rusting, corrosion, bending, breakage, and wear over time. However, with repeated use and processing, these tools may fail. The edges and points of surgical instruments can become dull, screws and ratchet mechanisms loosen, and precise opposing surfaces separate. As such, surgical instruments must be treated with care, inspected during the cleaning process, and repaired or replaced as necessary.

When an assistant hands an instrument to the surgeon, it is given handle first. This allows the surgeon to immediately use the instrument and also prevents injury from sharp parts of the tools. Similarly, when returning instruments back to the scrub tech, they are passed handle first. There are a multitude of instruments that can be used in surgery. For the purposes of this book, the most commonly used instruments will be discussed here.

FORCEPS

Surgical forceps, also known as graspers or pickups, are primarily used to grasp tissue in a quick and nimble manner. They are held between the surgeon's thumb and forefinger as one would hold a pencil, and are operated by opposing these fingers together to close the tips of the instrument (Fig. 5.1). They are constructed with a built-in memory so that in the resting state, the tips are a fixed distance apart. When operating the forceps, the tips are squeezed together and will grasp tissue. When pressure is taken off the tips, they will move back to the original separated configuration.

In addition to tissue, graspers are used to manipulate needles, such as after being passed through tissue. They can also be used to remove debris such as suture, errant clips, and clot from the operative field. They are precise instruments that allow delicate and small structures to be grasped in a wide gamut of spaces. Forceps come in a variety of lengths and widths, and may be either toothed or non-toothed. Surgical-grade graspers should oppose well, and those instruments with teeth should interlock smoothly.

Adson forceps (Fig. 5.2). Most commonly used to apply dressings such as Steri-Strips, these forceps can also be used to hold delicate skin or other tissue when suturing. They have a spring tension shank and are notable by their wide, flat thumb and forefinger grasping area. The tip of an Adson forceps tapers down to a narrow, short tip.

Adson forceps with teeth (Fig. 5.3). A variation of the Adson forceps, these are more commonly used to grasp skin. The teeth dig into the skin, allowing force when manipulating tissue. There are typically two teeth on one side of the instrument that interlock with one tooth on the other side.

Brown-Adson forceps (Fig. 5.4). These forceps are another variation of the Adson forceps that are used to grasp skin. They have multiple rows of teeth along the tip. A common configuration includes nine rows of two teeth on each side of the instrument that interlock when closed.

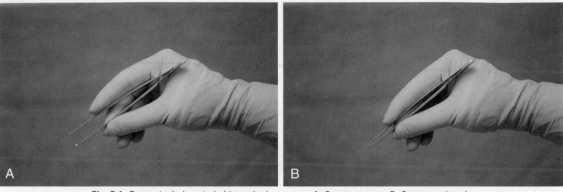

Fig. 5.1 Proper technique to hold surgical graspers. A. Graspers open. B. Graspers closed.

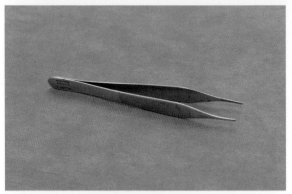

Fig. 5.2 Adson forceps

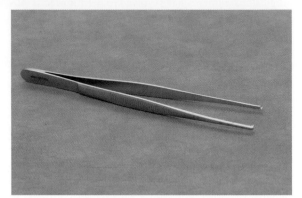

Fig. 5.5 Tissue forceps with teeth

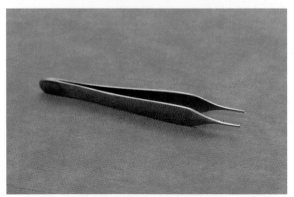

Fig. 5.3 Adson forceps with teeth

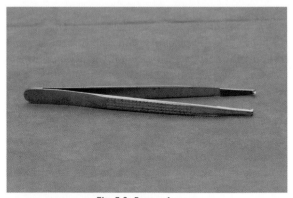

Fig. 5.6 Bonney forceps

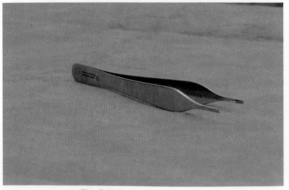

Fig. 5.4 Brown-Adson forceps

Tissue forceps with teeth (Fig. 5.5). Also known as adult forceps with teeth or thumb forceps with teeth, these are used to hold a variety of tissue types. The teeth are larger than those found on Adson forceps and generally are longer and narrower. They come with spring tension shanks and are available in a wide variety of lengths and widths. The width and opening of the tip ultimately dictates the thickness of tissue that can be grasped and manipulated with these forceps.

Bonney forceps (Fig. 5.6). These are heavy forceps ideally suited for grasping thick tissue such as

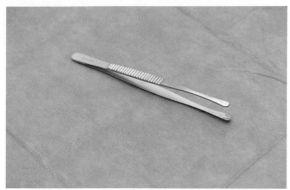

Fig. 5.7 Russian forceps

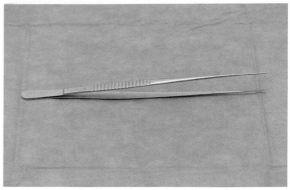

Fig. 5.9 DeBakey forceps

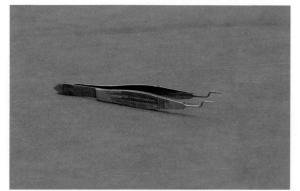

Fig. 5.8 Bayonet Cushing forceps with teeth

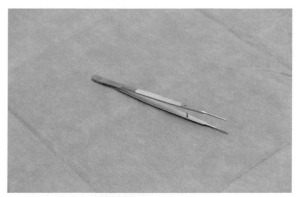

Fig. 5.10 Gerald forceps

fascia or bone. Although they are available both with and without teeth, Bonney forceps with teeth are more commonly used. They should not be used to grasp delicate tissue such as the bowel.

Russian forceps (Fig. 5.7). These are also moderately heavy forceps with a rounded, spoon-shaped tip containing radial serrations around the outside. They may be used during wound closure or to gain good purchase on moderately delicate tissue such as lymphatic tissue. Although the serrations on the tip of these forceps provide good holding strength on tissue, they are still relatively atraumatic. As with other types of forceps, they are available in a variety of lengths for different applications.

Cushing forceps (Fig. 5.8). These are relatively narrow-handled forceps available with or without teeth and used for fine dissection, commonly in neurosurgical cases. They are optimal for grasping delicate tissue or small suture and needles. Cushing forceps are available in both straight and bayonet configurations. The bayonet design offsets the surgeon's hands from the field of view.

DeBakey forceps (Fig. 5.9). This is one of the most commonly used forceps for grasping delicate tissue and

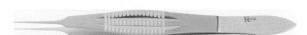

Fig. 5.11 Castroviejo forceps. Reproduced with permission from http://www.medline.com/media/mkt/pdf/Final-konig-PDF-Catalog.pdf

blood vessels during manipulation and suturing. These nontoothed forceps have fine jaws and are available in a multitude of lengths and jaw widths; however, they do not generate significant pressure at the tips to avoid traumatizing tissue. As such, they are not well suited for grasping thick or heavy tissue.

Gerald forceps (Fig. 5.10). These are a lightweight toothed or nontoothed tissue forceps similar to the DeBakey forceps; however, they have much narrower tips than DeBakey forceps and are only suited for grasping light, delicate tissue. They also often have a stop peg to prevent excessive crushing force on tissue.

Castroviejo forceps (Fig. 5.11). These are small forceps used for microsurgical procedures, most often in ophthalmology, plastic surgery, and delicate vascular anastomosis. They are shorter in length and have a locking mechanism between the tongs. They are designed to atraumatically hold tissue and small suture.

CLAMPS AND CLAMPING

Like forceps, surgical clamps are also intended to hold tissue; however, they differ in that they contain a locking mechanism to maintain a constant grip. The locking system is usually a ratchet on the shank of the instrument. This allows pressure at the tip to be applied iteratively, and an audible click is heard as the lock engages each ratchet (see Video 5.1). Most clamps also contain finger loops that facilitate their handling and placement. The loops are useful in both moving the clamps and releasing the locking mechanism. Clamps are differentiated by their tips, each being useful for grasping specific types of tissue. Clamps also can be used to hold various materials during surgery (suture, gauze pads, etc.). As with forceps, they may be toothed or nontoothed and are available in a wide variety of lengths, widths, and weights.

When a clamp is handed to a surgeon, the ratchet should be closed to prevent injury by the tips of the instrument. Again, the scrub tech should ensure that the instrument is passed to the surgeon so that the finger loops are in the palm of his hand and the instrument is ready for use. To hold a clamp, the surgeon places his thumb and fourth (ring) finger through the finger loops of the handle. The third (middle) finger is placed next to the adjacent finger loop. The index finger is placed along the shank of the instrument and is used to help stabilize it (Fig. 5.12). With experience, surgeons can operate the instrument with the palm of the hand, which is referred to as palming the instrument (Fig. 5.13). This can allow for quicker release and finer motion as the tool is operated closer to the tips.

Most surgical clamps are manufactured as "right-handed" clamps. To open these clamps with one's right hand, the thumb is used to press on its finger loop while the other finger loop is pulled by the fourth finger in the opposite direction. When opening these clamps with one's left hand, the thumb finger loop is pulled while the opposite finger loop is pushed to release the ratchet mechanism (see Video 5.1).

Mosquito clamp (also known as Crile, Pean, Rochester, stat, or snap) (Fig. 5.14). These clamps are relatively short instruments with fine tips and can be either curved or straight. They are easily distinguished from other clamps by their short and serrated jaws that interdigitate when closed. Mosquitos can be used as hemostatic forceps (hemostat), clamping delicate blood vessels so that they can be ligated or cauterized. Additionally, they can be used to hold delicate tissue or the ends of suture material prior to the sutures being cut. When using a mosquito for this purpose, the tip of the instrument, as opposed to the middle of the jaws, should be used to grasp the suture.

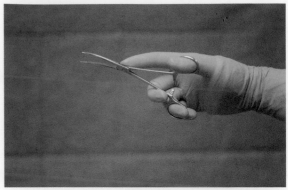
Fig. 5.12 The proper way to hold a surgical clamp

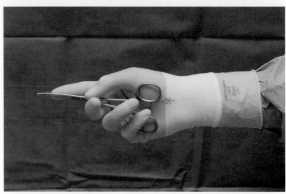
Fig. 5.13 Palming an instrument

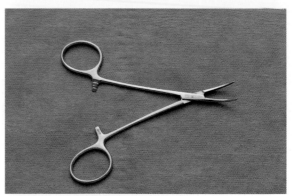
Fig. 5.14 Curved mosquito clamp

Kelly clamp (Fig. 5.15). The handle of these clamps is longer and heavier than mosquito clamps. They also have longer interdigitated serrated jaws that are blunt at the tip. They can be either straight or curved. Kelly clamps are useful for grasping larger blood vessels or tissue to be sutured, ligated, or cauterized. Additionally, they can be used to dissect soft tissue by spreading the jaws open. For example, Kelly clamps are often chosen to dissect through subcutaneous tissue.

Kocher clamp (Fig. 5.16). These clamps are medium-large instruments used to grasp heavy tissue such

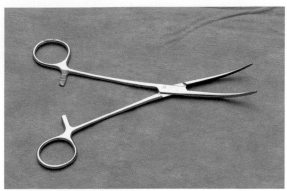

Fig. 5.15 Kelly clamp

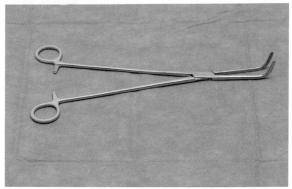

Fig. 5.18 Carmalt clamp

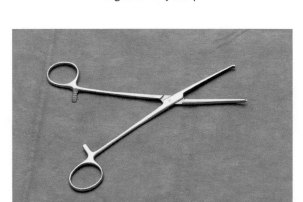

Fig. 5.16 Kocher clamp

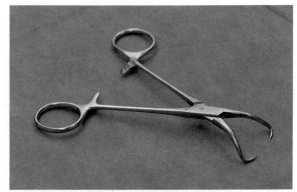

Fig. 5.19 Backhaus towel clamp

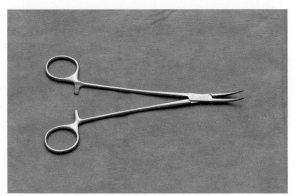

Fig. 5.17 Tonsil clamp

as fascia. They may be either curved or straight, although straight Kocher clamps are more commonly used. They have horizontally serrated tips and heavy teeth at the tip of the instrument, both of which provide excellent holding strength on tissue. One should be careful not to grab bowel or other delicate tissue with these instruments, as the teeth will cause a perforation and with tension can tear tissue.

Tonsil clamp (Fig. 5.17). These instruments derive their name from their use in placing packing or holding sponges for tonsillectomy procedures. They contain

short and fine, serrated, curved tips without teeth. They may also be used for fine dissection of soft tissues.

Carmalt clamp (Fig. 5.18). These hemostatic forceps are distinguishable by their longitudinally serrated curved or straight jaws that contain horizontal serrations at the tips. The horizontal serrations allow this clamp to provide better holding strength on tissue as the instrument is lifted in a plane parallel to the length of the clamp.

Backhaus towel clamp (Fig. 5.19). Often referred to simply as a towel clamp, these instruments were designed to secure drapes and towels together when draping a patient. They contain very sharp perforating prongs that oppose when closed. The towel clamp can also be used to grasp and manipulate tissue and bone by perforating the tissue.

Nonperforating towel clamp (Fig. 5.20). This clamp is similar to a Backhaus towel clamp, although as its name suggests, it does not perforate tissue. For this reason, these clamps are safer than ordinary towel clamps but may not hold draping material together as well. The tips of these instruments are either round or square and may contain serrations.

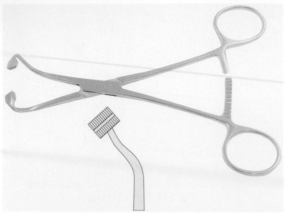

Fig. 5.20 Nonperforating towel clamp. Reproduced with permission from http://www.medline.com/media/mkt/pdf/Final-konig-PDF-Catalog.pdf

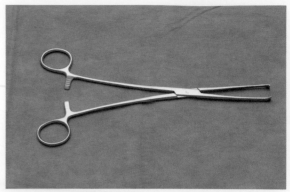

Fig. 5.22 Allis tissue clamp

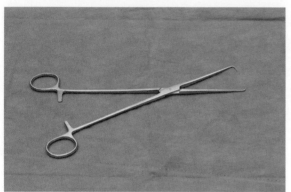

Fig. 5.21 Tenaculum clamp

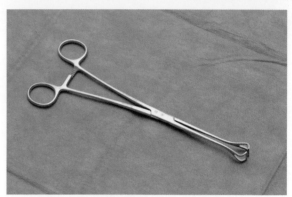

Fig. 5.23 Babcock tissue clamp

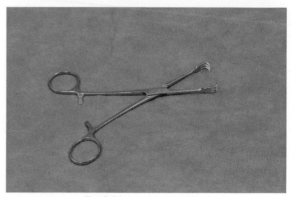

Fig. 5.24 Lahey goiter clamp

Tenaculum clamp (Fig. 5.21). This clamp contains a pair of sharp opposing prongs at the tip of the instrument, which are ideal for firmly grasping thick, dense tissue or masses and allow for manipulation of the tissue. Tenaculum clamps are commonly used to grasp and manipulate the uterus or masses of the breast. Although they do perforate tissue, they do not crush it, making them ideal for grasping tissue that will undergo pathologic evaluation.

Allis tissue clamp (Fig. 5.22). This clamp is long and thin, and is distinguished by its tip, which is perpendicular to the rest of the jaws. Along the tip is a row of interlocking teeth. The main body of the jaws themselves do not oppose, but the tips do. Allis clamps are used to grasp delicate and slippery tissue with minimal trauma to the tissue itself. They are often used to grasp breast and vaginal tissue, as well as open intestinal edges.

Babcock tissue clamp (Fig. 5.23). Like the Allis clamp, this clamp is long and thin with opposing tips that are perpendicular to the main body of the jaws. The tips themselves are atraumatic and therefore are useful for grasping delicate tissue.

They have a fenestrated opening at the tips of the jaws as opposed to a solid body, making them more delicate when closed and preventing crush injuries to delicate structures. Babcock clamps are also very useful for circumscribing and controlling tubular structures such as blood vessels and the ureters.

Lahey goiter clamp (Fig. 5.24). This clamp is constructed with three opposing prongs on each side of the instrument tip that are used to penetrate and grasp tissue. Similar to a tenaculum clamp, the prongs penetrate tissue but do not crush it. They are

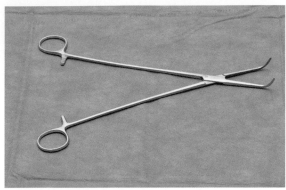

Fig. 5.25 Right-angle clamp

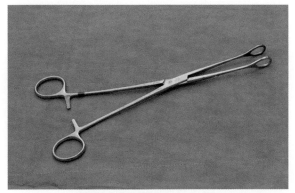

Fig. 5.26 Foerster sponge clamp

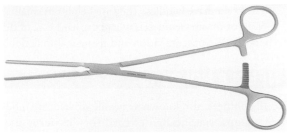

Fig. 5.27 Glover clamp. Reproduced with permission from http://www.medline.com/media/mkt/pdf/Final-konig-PDF-Catalog.pdf

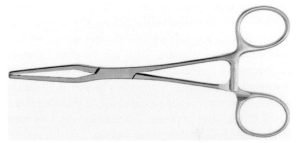

Fig. 5.28 Fogarty clamp. Reproduced with permission from http://www.medline.com/media/mkt/pdf/Final-konig-PDF-Catalog.pdf

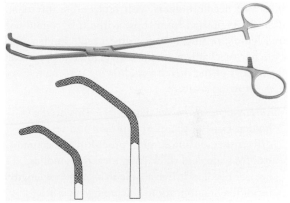

Fig. 5.29 Satinsky clamp. Reproduced with permission from http://www.medline.com/media/mkt/pdf/Final-konig-PDF-Catalog.pdf

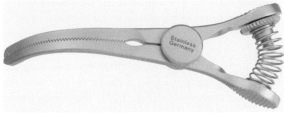

Fig. 5.30 Bulldog clamp. Reproduced with permission from http://www.medline.com/media/mkt/pdf/Final-konig-PDF-Catalog.pdf

typically used to grasp and manipulate heavy, firm tissue.

Right-angle clamp (also known as the Mixter or Rienhoff clamp) (Fig. 5.25). These clamps are distinguished by their fully serrated, right-angle tips. They are available in multiple lengths as well as the acuteness of the right-angle curve. Whereas some are fully curved to 90 degrees, others have a more obtuse angle curve. They are useful for clamping, grasping, and dissecting tissue in small spaces that would otherwise be inaccessible with straight instruments. The offset tip allows the surgeon to dissect under direct vision. The Rienhoff version has a gentler bend in the neck and again is helpful in dissection.

Foerster sponge clamp (Fig. 5.26). This clamp, also known as a sponge-holding forceps or a sponge stick, is used to hold a folded sponge for dissection or for absorbing fluid in the surgical field. The tips are oval shaped with serrations and contain a fenestration in the middle.

Vascular clamps [Glover (Fig. 5.27), Fogarty (Fig. 5.28), Satinsky (Fig. 5.29), Bulldog (Fig. 5.30)]. These are a family of clamps that can be placed across large vessels, such as the iliac arteries or vena cava. They have noncrushing tips that oppose

evenly over a relatively long surface area and come in straight, right-angled, and curved varieties. Satinsky clamps have a characteristic C-shaped tip that can be used for side biting or tangentially occluding a vessel. Bulldog clamps are detachable spring-loaded clamps that do not have handles. They are helpful in small spaces or on smaller vessels where the hardware of the handles may obscure vision and tissue manipulation.

NEEDLE HOLDERS

Needle holders, also known as needle drivers, are modified clamps, specifically designed for the purpose of throwing sutures. They come in a variety of weights and lengths, as well as curvature of the tip. Most needle drivers are ring handled, although some surgeons prefer to not place their fingers in the rings and instead palm the handle of the needle driver. The jaws of most needle drivers are smaller and shorter, albeit thicker, than most other clamps. They can be either smooth or serrated. Whereas smooth jaws minimize damage to the needle, serrated jaws provide a greater hold on the needle. Because of their repeated use in grasping metal needles, the jaws of these instruments tend to wear faster than those of other instruments. For this reason, some needle holders contain replaceable jaw inserts designed to extend the overall life of the instrument. These inserts are usually constructed of tungsten-carbide, and needle holders with replaceable inserts are often distinguished from those without by a gold-colored handle or finger rings. Most needle holders have a ratchet mechanism useful for stabilizing the needle in the jaws of the driver, yet allowing it to be released after throwing a suture.

Mayo-Hegar needle holder (Fig. 5.31). This needle holder is one of the most common and versatile drivers used during surgical procedures. It contains stubby, wide, and thick jaws, ideal for handling heavier needles. It is available in a variety of lengths for different applications, including superficial suturing and suturing in deep spaces.

Webster needle holder (Fig. 5.32). This is a commonly used needle holder for smaller needles and finer suture material. It is a short driver that allows for precise control of the needle and is therefore often used in plastic surgery and for subcutaneous suturing applications. The jaws of this driver may either be serrated or smooth, with selection based on surgeon preference and the degree of needle control required.

Crile-Wood needle holder (Fig. 5.33). This needle holder features short stubby jaws, with a gently tapered, blunt tip. It is more delicate than Mayo-Hegar needle holders but less delicate than Webster needle holders. It is available with either smooth or cross-serrated jaws.

Olsen-Hegar needle holder (Fig. 5.34). This needle holder features a built-in cutting edge just proximal to the tip of the instrument. It is useful when performing interrupted sutures, allowing the surgeon

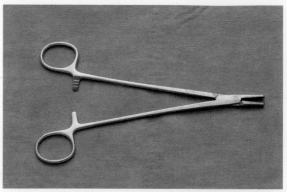

Fig. 5.31 Mayo-Hegar needle holder

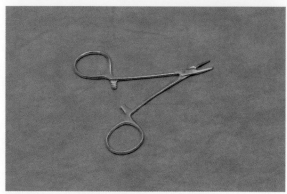

Fig. 5.32 Webster needle holder

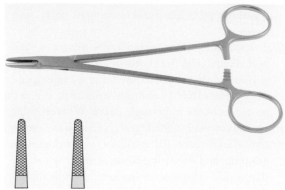

Fig. 5.33 Crile-Wood needle holder. Reproduced with permission from http://www.medline.com/media/mkt/pdf/Final-konig-PDF-Catalog.pdf

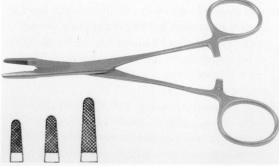

Fig. 5.34 Olsen-Hegar needle holder. Reproduced with permission from http://www.medline.com/media/mkt/pdf/Final-konig-PDF-Catalog.pdf

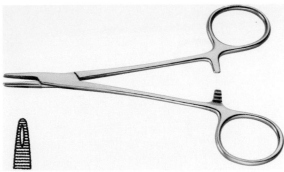

Fig. 5.35 Collier needle holder. Reproduced with permission from http://www.medline.com/media/mkt/pdf/Final-konig-PDF-Catalog.pdf

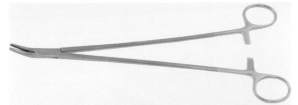

Fig. 5.37 Finochietto needle holder. Reproduced with permission from http://www.medline.com/media/mkt/pdf/Final-konig-PDF-Catalog.pdf

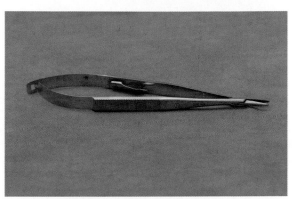

Fig. 5.38 Castroviejo needle holder

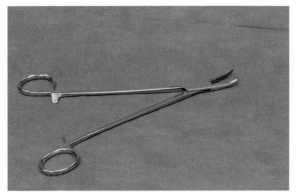

Fig. 5.36 Heaney needle holder

to quickly cut suture without switching instruments. The needle-holding jaws of the instrument are cross serrated.

Collier needle holder (Fig. 5.35). This needle holder contains serrations and has fenestrated jaws. It is typically used for delicate suturing, ideally suited to hold 3-0, 4-0, or 5-0 suture material.

Heaney needle holder (Fig. 5.36). This needle holder is distinguished by its slightly curved jaws, making it ideal for suturing in narrow spaces. It is commonly used for intravaginal suturing with light to medium weight suture material and needles. The jaws of this driver contain cross serrations.

Finochietto needle holder (Fig. 5.37). Similar to the Heaney needle driver, this needle driver has an angled tip and typically a long shank, and is useful for suturing in narrow and deep spaces. It is therefore ideal for Ob/Gyn procedures and when performing colorectal anastomoses.

Castroviejo needle holder (Fig. 5.38). This needle driver has thin jaws and is designed for delicate suturing with small, fine needles. It is distinguished by its spring handle, as opposed to the typical ratchet mechanism, and has a lock or catch to hold the needle. It does not contain finger rings and is instead opened and closed by opposing the thumb

and index finger. From a closed position, depressing the shank of the instrument opens it with a click. To close it, the shank is pressed again until it clicks, locking the jaws in a closed position.

SCISSORS

Scissors are used for dissection and to cut tissue, suture material, and supplies during surgical cases. Most types of scissors are available in a variety of lengths and may come with straight, angled, or curved cutting surfaces. Scissors may be either sharp or blunt at the tip depending on their application and intended use. It is important to remember that, as with other surgical instruments, scissors are delicate, and each type should be used only for its intended purpose. As such, scissors specifically designed to cut suture material should not be used to cut tissue, and scissors that are designed for dissection should not be used to cut suture material or other supplies. They need to be regularly maintained and sharpened to preserve their sharp cutting surfaces.

Mayo scissors (Fig. 5.39). This is one of the most versatile and commonly used surgical scissors. They are relatively thick and can therefore be used to cut through tough, thick tissue or suture material. Mayo scissors are available in a large variety of lengths. The tips of these scissors have a beveled blade and blunt tips, and may be either straight or curved.

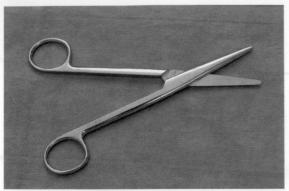

Fig. 5.39 Straight Mayo scissors

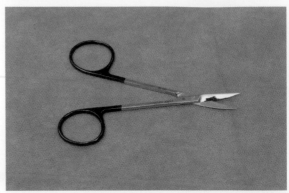

Fig. 5.41 Curved Iris scissors.

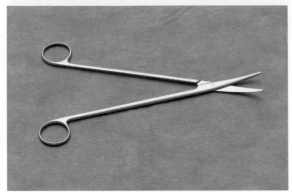

Fig. 5.40 Curved Metzenbaum (Metz) scissors

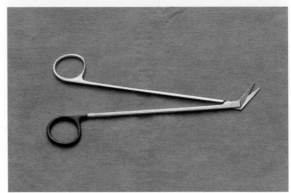

Fig. 5.42 Potts-Smith scissors

Metzenbaum (Metz) scissors (Fig. 5.40). One of the most commonly used dissecting scissors, Metzenbaum scissors are specifically designed to cut and dissect tissue and should not be used to cut suture material or supplies. These scissors have blunt tips, are available in variety of lengths, and can be either straight or curved.

Iris scissors (Fig. 5.41). These scissors derive their name from their original use in ophthalmologic procedures. They contain a fine tip with a sharp point and may be either curved, angled, or straight. They are often used for detailed dissection of tissue.

Potts-Smith scissors (Fig. 5.42). These scissors are specifically used for delicate dissection of soft tissues. They have a short, very sharply pointed tip and are available in different tip angles, including 25, 45, and 60 degrees. They are commonly used for trimming delicate tissue and blood vessels, as well as opening vessels and tubular structures.

Stevens tenotomy scissors (Fig. 5.43). These scissors are used for delicate dissection and cutting. They contain sharp blades with fine, sharply pointed tips and relatively long handles for control. They are available in both straight and curved configurations.

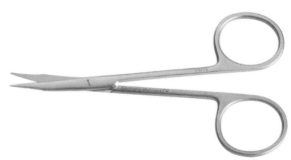

Fig. 5.43 Curved Stevens tenotomy scissors. Used with permission from Medline.

Westcott tenotomy scissors (Fig. 5.44). These scissors are similar to Stevens tenotomy scissors in use and tip configuration, except they have a spring handle and do not have finger loops. They are operated similarly to the Castroviejo needle holder; however, they do not have a catch. Therefore, when closed, they will spring open automatically.

Lister bandage scissors (Fig. 5.45). These scissors are commonly used for sizing dressings, cutting plaster, and trimming bandages. They are heavy scissors with angled jaws. The lower jaw has a blunt probe

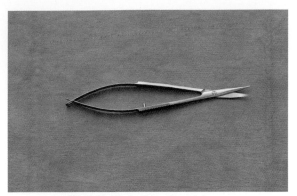

Fig. 5.44 Westcott tenotomy scissors

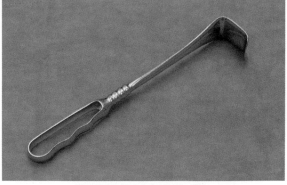

Fig. 5.46 Richardson retractor

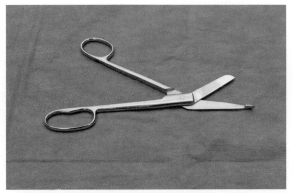

Fig. 5.45 Lister bandage scissors

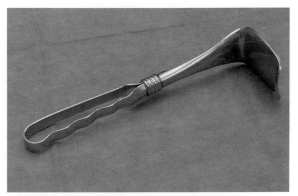

Fig. 5.47 Kelly retractor

at the tip and is usually longer than the upper jaw. This configuration makes the lower jaw useful for sliding between the skin and a dressing without causing injury to the skin.

RETRACTORS AND RETRACTING

Surgical retractors serve to hold an incision open to provide exposure to the surgical field. A variety of shapes and sizes are available depending on the application. They may be handheld or self-retaining, as well as fixed in shape or malleable. The type and quality of retraction can drive the size of an incision.

Handheld Retractors

Handheld retractors allow the working side of the instrument to be placed within the incision and positioned to offer exposure to the surgical wound. These retractors typically have a curved, hooked, or angled blade. The opposite side of the retractor usually contains a handle that an assistant may use to draw back on the instrument, thereby opening the wound. The handles are long enough to keep an assistant's hands out of the way of the surgeon.

Richardson retractor (Fig. 5.46). This retractor is commonly used to hold the edges of an abdominal

incision open. It is available in multiple sizes to provide adequate retraction without being too bulky. The blade is slightly concave, configured at a right angle, and contains blunt edges. This configuration allows it to catch under the edge of an incision and draw back multiple layers of tissue. The handle contains multiple ridges for a comfortable grip.

Kelly retractor (Fig. 5.47). This retractor is very similar to a standard Richardson retractor with a slightly concave, right-angle blade. It is therefore often referred to as a Kelly Richardson. However, it is distinguished from a standard Richardson retractor in that it contains a longer blade.

Deaver retractor (Fig. 5.48). This retractor, shaped like a question mark, contains a thin, flat blade that is less rigid than the blade of a Richardson retractor. It may have a grip handle similar to that found on a Richardson retractor or a flat handle that can be clamped for use in a self-retaining retractor, such as a Bookwalter retractor. These come in various widths and are used for retracting organs, as the interface surface is smooth.

Harrington (sweetheart) retractor (Fig. 5.49). This retractor is designed for retraction of organs deep in the abdominal cavity. The tip of the curved blade of

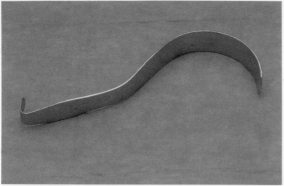

Fig. 5.48 Deaver retractor

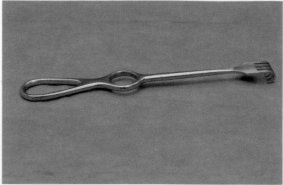

Fig. 5.51 Volkmann (rake) retractor

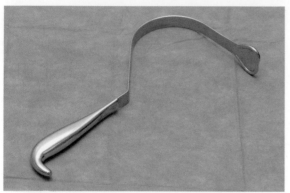

Fig. 5.49 Harrington (sweetheart) retractor

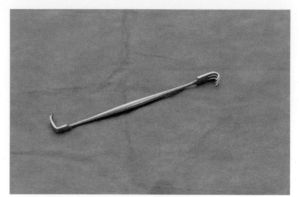

Fig. 5.52 Senn retractor

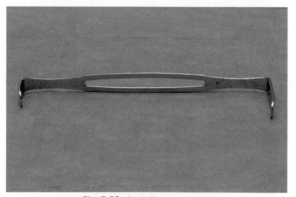

Fig. 5.50 Army-Navy retractor

this instrument resembles that of a heart, reducing trauma to organs such as the spleen and liver. It also contains a grip handle.

Army-Navy retractor (Fig. 5.50). This is a dual-ended rigid retractor in which one blade is longer than the other. The blades are oriented at a 90-degree angle with a slight curve at the tip of the blade and are of a fixed size. Army-Navy retractors are often used as a set to pull and hold the edges of a superficial wound apart.

Volkmann (rake) retractor (Fig. 5.51). The blade of this retractor is generally configured with one to six

sharp or blunt prongs oriented at a right angle to the handle of the instrument. Volkmann retractors are commonly used to hold very superficial tissue apart and are popular for use in moving the skin during orthopedic joint procedures.

Senn retractor (Fig. 5.52). This dual-ended retractor contains a right-angle, blunt blade at one end and a blunt or sharp-tip three-prong configuration at the other end. Senn retractors are often used for superficial tissue retraction, holding the edges of a wound apart.

Cushing vein retractor (Fig. 5.53). This retractor has a narrow handle and contains an aggressively curved blade. It is useful for cradling delicate structures such as veins and nerves. It is small enough to fit into deep, narrow spaces for retraction of blood vessels and nerves.

Ribbon (malleable) retractor (Fig. 5.54). This retractor, as its name suggests, is constructed of flexible steel that can be shaped as necessary to fit into multiple spaces and with myriad different configurations. It is available in a variety of lengths and widths, and it can be clamped for use as part of a self-retaining retractor system. It can also be placed inside of an incision during wound closure to prevent injury to underlying structures such as bowel.

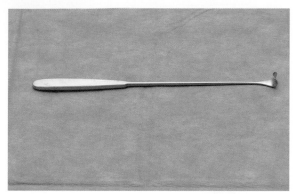

Fig. 5.53 Cushing vein retractor

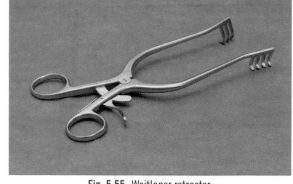

Fig. 5.55 Weitlaner retractor

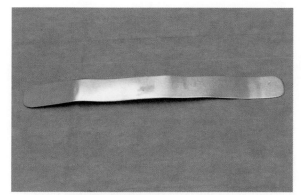

Fig. 5.54 Ribbon (malleable) retractor

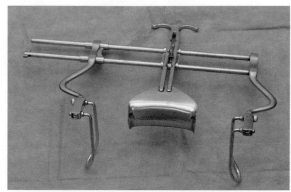

Fig. 5.56 Balfour retractor with center blade attached

Self-Retaining Retractors

Self-retaining retractors are placed in a surgical wound to help keep the wound open without physical assistance. They do so by using a self-contained ratcheting or spring mechanism, or by allowing opposing instruments to pull against each other and the wound edges. Self-retaining retractors come in sizes that allow for exposure to both small and large wounds.

Weitlaner retractor (Fig. 5.55). This self-retaining retractor is designed for use on relatively small incisions. It utilizes a ratchet lock mechanism, in which the opposing sides of the instrument are locked apart. Each side contains between two and six outward-curving blunt or sharp prong tips that when spread apart provide grip for retention and traction to hold an incision open.

Balfour retractor (Fig. 5.56). This self-retaining retractor is predominantly used in laparotomy procedures. It contains two outward-curving solid or fenestrated blades that are placed within an incision and spread open to hold the wound edges apart. It is important to place moistened laparotomy sponges between the blades of the retractor and the incision to prevent dehydration and injury to the sides of the incision. This retractor allows for a variety of additional blades to be attached to the rail in

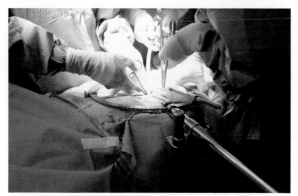

Fig. 5.57 Bookwalter retractor system

the center of the instrument to provide additional exposure to the wound.

Bookwalter retractor (Fig. 5.57). The Bookwalter retractor is a highly modifiable retractor system. Whereas other self-retaining retractors spread the incision apart and are held in place by the opposing force of the incision, the Bookwalter system requires it to be anchored to the operating table by a clamp. This clamp is attached to a bar that projects vertically to a level above the patient. A post coupling clamp is used to attach a horizontal bar to the table bar. Attached to this is a ring, typically in the shape

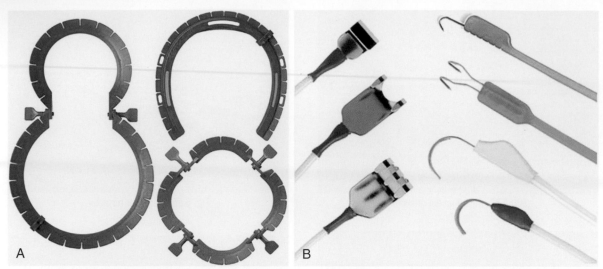

Fig. 5.58 Lone Star retractor system. A. Lone Star self-retaining retractors. Reproduced with permission from http://www.coopersurgical.com/Products/Detail/Lone-Star-Disposable-Retractors. B. Lone Star self-retaining retractor stays. Reproduced with permission from http://www.coopersurgical.com/Products/Detail/Lone-Star-Elastic-Stays

of a circle or oval, which is positioned above the incision. Various blades can then be attached to the ring and placed within the incision to hold it open. These are attached to the ring via either a clamp with a ratchet used to tilt the blade or a nontilting clamp.

Lone Star retractor (Fig. 5.58). This self-retaining retractor is available as either a stainless steel reusable retractor or as a plastic disposable system. It is primarily used for smaller incisions on the perineum or on the head. The retractor itself is positioned over an incision and allows for stays to be positioned in the wound and fixed to the body of the retractor. Typically a stay placed within the wound is opposed by another stay that pulls the edge of the wound open in the opposite direction. Stays can be blunt or sharp-tipped single prongs, or a rake. The body of the retractor is available in different shapes, including an oval, a circle, or a square configuration.

CAUTERY DEVICES

Cautery is used in nearly all surgical procedures, from a simple excision of a skin lesion to more complex abdominal cases. Cautery devices may be used to either cut or coagulate tissue, and most devices have the ability to perform both functions via separate controls. Some instruments perform cutting and coagulation functions simultaneously, although they often cannot be separated from each other. Additionally, many cautery devices are available as both handheld instruments with a rocker switch on the handle or for use as a laparoscopic instrument that is foot controlled.

When the cutting mode of an instrument is used, a high power density is applied to the tip of the instrument to vaporize tissue. However, this may result in bleeding if the instrument is used over a blood vessel, and as such does not provide hemostasis. The cutting function of a cautery device can be used to incise the superficial layers of skin or delicate tissue.

In contrast, the coagulation mode of an instrument uses a lower power density to generate thermal coagulation and can control bleeding. It is often used to proceed through subcutaneous skin layers and for the majority of surgical cautery applications, as it minimizes bleeding from small vessels. The coagulation mode of an instrument does have a tissue-destructive effect and therefore is not used to cut skin to minimize scarring. When activating cautery, there is an audible signal produced by the generator box. The tone produced differs when using cutting compared to coagulation modes and is activated as a safety signal to alert the surgeon as to which mode is active.

Energy may be delivered via either a monopolar or bipolar instrument, although in both cases a complete electrical circuit is required. Monopolar instruments work by delivering energy from a generator through an active electrode, which is the instrument itself. Energy is transmitted to the target tissue and is picked up by the dispersive electrode "grounding pad." It is then returned to the generator by the dispersive pad. Prior to draping, this pad must be placed on the patient for each type of cautery unit being used. For example, when a surgeon plans to use both a Bovie cautery pen and LigaSure device during a surgical procedure, grounding pads for each of these devices must be placed on the patient. However, because energy has the potential to

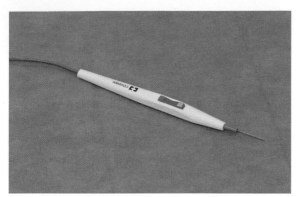

Fig. 5.59 Electrosurgical pencil

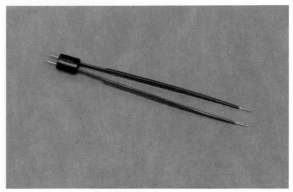

Fig. 5.60 Bipolar forceps

be dispersed to nearby tissues, caution needs to be used in patients who have implanted devices.

Bipolar instruments contain both electrodes within the instrument itself. Energy from a generator therefore only passes through the tissue contained between the two sides of the forceps. This allows the energy to be restricted to a much smaller area of tissue than when using monopolar instruments and is thus useful in patients with metal implants or when there is risk of damage to nearby structures. These devices have a limited ability to cauterize large areas and are generally effective primarily with minor bleeding.

Electrosurgical pencil (Fig. 5.59). Commonly referred to as a Bovie pencil after William Bovie, the first individual to develop and use an electrosurgical pencil, this instrument delivers monopolar energy to tissue. Held like a pencil, these instruments are operated with either the thumb or forefinger to deliver cutting or coagulating current to tissue. They may be placed directly on the tissue to be cauterized or coupled to another metal instrument such as a forceps or laparoscopic instrument to deliver energy. These instruments may be disposable or reusable, although they always utilize a disposable tip. The tip itself may be a narrow spatula or a fine needle point.

Bipolar forceps (Fig. 5.60). These are highly precise instruments that are used to grasp and deliver bipolar energy to tissue. They usually contain a spring tension shank and are held between the thumb and forefinger as one would hold a forceps. They are excellent at providing energy only to the tissue between the tips of the forceps and are therefore utilized when the delivery of concentrated, precise energy is necessary.

LigaSure device (Fig. 5.61). This device is available for both open and laparoscopic applications, and is utilized to both seal and cut tissue. The jaws of the device are placed around the selected tissue. By squeezing the handle, the jaws of the device are

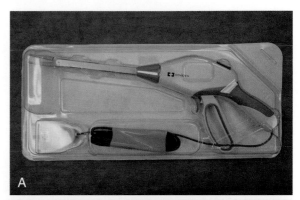

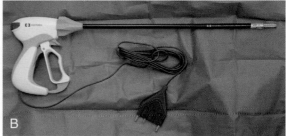

Fig. 5.61 LigaSure device. A. LigaSure open surgical device. © Ethicon 2017. Reproduced with permission. B. LigaSure laparoscopic surgical device. © Ethicon 2017. Reproduced with permission.

locked in the closed position around the tissue. Activation of the instrument delivers energy to the tissue and cauterizes it. At the end of the cycle, a beep alerts the user that adequate tissue seal has occurred. By activating the trigger of the instrument, the tissue is cut in the middle of where it was sealed. Squeezing the handle a second time unlocks the jaws of the instrument. This device has the potential to seal and cut large pieces of tissue as well as blood vessels up to 8 mm.

Harmonic scalpel (Fig. 5.62). This instrument is an alternative to the LigaSure device and also is available as both an open and laparoscopic instrument. Like the LigaSure, it serves to seal and cut tissue. It accomplishes this simultaneously, however,

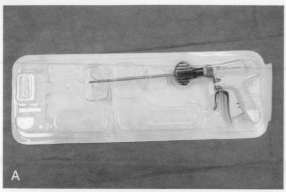
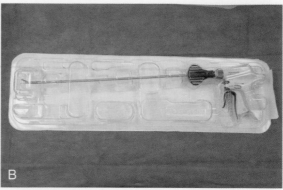

Fig. 5.62 Harmonic scalpel. A. Open instrument. B. Laparoscopic instrument.

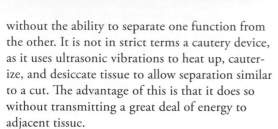

Fig. 5.63 Laparoscopic argon beam coagulator

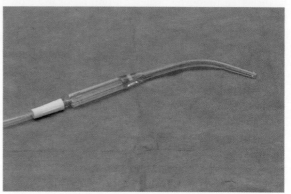

Fig. 5.64 Yankauer suction tip

without the ability to separate one function from the other. It is not in strict terms a cautery device, as it uses ultrasonic vibrations to heat up, cauterize, and desiccate tissue to allow separation similar to a cut. The advantage of this is that it does so without transmitting a great deal of energy to adjacent tissue.

Argon beam coagulator (Fig. 5.63). This device, available as both a handheld and laparoscopic instrument, is used for creating superficial hemostasis. A stream of argon gas is emitted from the tip of the instrument, and an electrical charge is applied to the gas. This results in a short spray of electricity that causes cauterization to a depth of 1 to 2 mm. The advantage of this is that it can provide hemostasis without touching the tissue itself and is useful for the oozing surfaces of delicate solid organs such as that of the liver, spleen, and kidney. It is not meant for sealing larger vessels.

SUCTION DEVICES

Suction devices are used to keep the surgical field clear of blood and bodily fluids, irrigation fluids placed in the surgical wound, and smoke. Wall suction provides negative pressure and is connected to a suction canister

via tubing where the fluid is collected for safe disposal. From the canister, sterile tubing is run to the surgical field and connected to a hand-piece suction tip. This suction tip provides suction at the level of the wound. Suction tips can be either disposable or reusable.

Yankauer suction tip (Fig. 5.64). This is the most commonly used suction tip for surgical procedures. It is typically constructed of a plastic hand piece with a gently curved shaft, although it may also be made of surgical stainless steel. The tip of the instrument contains a blunt bulbous head with one or more openings to allow for suction of fluids. The atraumatic design of this suction tip prevents inadvertent injury to surrounding tissue while providing effective suction.

Poole suction tip (Fig. 5.65). This suction tip is usually constructed of a hand piece with a straight shaft. It contains multiple small pores at the end of the hand piece that allows pooled blood and other fluids to be evacuated from deep abdominal wounds. It can also easily be converted to a pinpoint suction device by twisting the hand piece to expose an inner nonporous shaft.

Frazier suction tip (Fig. 5.66). This suction tip is used for fine, delicate suctioning applications. A thin

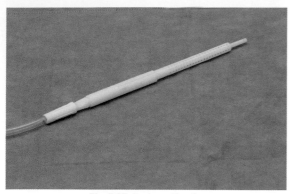

Fig. 5.65 Poole suction tip

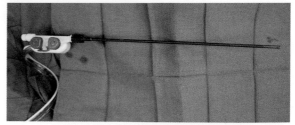

Fig. 5.67 Laparoscopic suction device

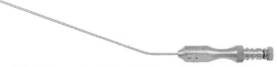

Fig. 5.66 Frazier suction tip. Used with permission from Medline.

curved metal shaft with a single opening at the end provides suction from the hand piece. An opening more proximally located on the instrument may also be used to regulate suctioning by the instru-

ment. When a surgeon places a finger over the opening, this allows the suction to draw fluid and debris from the field. When the finger is moved, air is drawn in through the opening and suction from the tip of the instrument ceases.

Laparoscopic suction device (Fig. 5.67). This suction tip is attached to a disposable suction irrigator with preattached tubing. The device allows a surgeon to simultaneously irrigate a wound and rapidly provide suction with the same instrument. After being placed through a laparoscopic port site, pressing the blue button on the suction irrigator allows the surgeon to irrigate a wound, whereas pressing the red button provides suction.

CHAPTER 6

ASSISTING IN THE OR: HOW TO HELP AND NOT GET IN THE WAY

Surgery is a coordinated, choreographed process. To avoid chaos and assure optimal outcomes, each individual working at the operative field has a defined role. The surgeon sets out the plan and determines the rhythm and cadence of the procedure. She should effectively communicate all necessary needs and steps with the entire operating room (OR) team.

Assistants perform many integral roles during the course of an operation. Of these roles, one of the primary responsibilities of an assistant is to expose and keep the operative field clear for vision. As a surgeon has only two hands, the assistant may be needed to incise, tie, or manipulate tissue exposed by the surgeon. The assistant's firsthand involvement allows him to prepare for the next steps of an operation and to subtly communicate with the scrub tech when the surgeon is deeply focused on a technical issue.

The scrub tech is responsible for keeping order in the sterile field, tracking instruments and supplies, and providing equipment to the surgeon and assistants. The tech also anticipates needs in the operating field and communicates with the circulator, who can retrieve required equipment.

The nursing staff coordinates and documents operational activities. They gather equipment, coordinate and track supply movement in the room, communicate with staff outside the OR, and document the procedure.

The anesthesia team is tasked with anesthetizing patients, monitoring physiologic status, and maintaining homeostasis. Anesthesia providers play a key role in patient positioning to prevent intraoperative injuries. They also are responsible for administering systemic medications mandated by each procedure, such as antibiotics and muscle relaxants.

There is an OR etiquette. The surgeon first chooses the side of the table on which he will stand. This is defined by numerous factors, including the type of procedure, surgeon handedness, and habitus of the patient on the table. The goal is to allow the surgeon optimal visualization of the operative field while at the same time giving his dominant hand access to perform required maneuvers. The first assistant often stands on the side of the table opposite that of the surgeon, whereas additional assistants are placed strategically to help with retraction and other responsibilities.

Most individuals progress in the OR from passive observers to active assistants to performing the most complex parts of a surgical case. This chapter focuses on the basic aspects of how to help in the OR, and although most principles discussed here are aimed at assisting in the OR, many can be applied to the role of the primary surgeon as well.

WHERE TO STAND

One of the most basic yet oftentimes bewildering questions a new participant in the OR may have is simply, "Where should I stand?" The answer to this question is often not as simple as it may seem and depends on several factors, including the type of case being performed, whether the individual is scrubbed and at the field, the number of other participants in the room and at the patient bedside, and the level of participation of that individual.

Individuals who are scrubbed should stay as close to the sterile field as possible to prevent contact with nonsterile individuals and equipment in the room. Scrubbed individuals should always keep their hands above their waists and above the patient table. It is acceptable to rest one's hands on the patient, outside of the immediate surgical wound; however, care should be taken to not lean on the patient, as this could result in patient injury.

Nonscrubbed Individuals

In general, individuals who are not scrubbed should maintain a safe distance from the field to prevent contaminating drapes, instruments, and scrubbed individuals. The ideal place for a nonscrubbed observer to stand is where he can adequately observe the surgery being performed without compromising sterility.

This will vary depending on the manner in which the surgery is being performed, as well as the specific type of surgery. Laparoscopic and endoscopic surgeries often afford observers the opportunity to see the surgery on a monitor as it is being performed. During these surgeries, observers are able to visualize the exact same thing a surgeon is seeing and are able to stand almost anywhere in the OR that a monitor is visible. Oftentimes it is most convenient to stay at the periphery of the room for this purpose. If possible, it may be valuable for a nonscrubbed individual to stand with a good view of the team. As such, he can also observe the surgeon, tech, and assistants to appreciate how the team works (Fig. 6.1).

In robotic cases, there are several options for optimal viewing. As with laparoscopic surgeries, video screens are available. A surgeon may allow an observer a view through the robotic console, as it is away from the operative field and not considered sterile. Some institutions have a dual-console robotic surgical system that allows nonscrubbed individuals the opportunity to visualize a surgery as it is being performed in three dimensions, assuming there is not a surgeon at the second console.

Open surgical cases can be challenging for a nonscrubbed observer to fully visualize the procedure. In ORs that have camera systems built into overhead lighting handles, individuals may still be able to observe the procedure on a monitor. This view is limited to where the light is positioned and may not always afford the same view of the surgeon and assistants. In many open cases, observers may need to switch between multiple different positions to view the surgery.

Utilization of standing stools allows both scrubbed and nonscrubbed personnel to obtain a higher viewpoint and see around the surgeon. Whereas taller individuals may be able to view a procedure over the shoulders of surgeons, most observers will gain a much better view via the use of a standing stool (Fig. 6.2). The anesthesia work area is usually the space at the head of the table, often flanked by IV poles that confine the drape. Once the patient is asleep and stable, the anesthesia team may allow a nonscrubbed individual to look over the drapes and view a procedure (Fig. 6.3). This is particularly helpful in abdominal, thoracic, and head and neck cases, which are closer to the head of the bed.

In all cases, the noise level should be kept to a minimum to facilitate communication in the OR. Some surgeons allow music that they feel helps pace the operation, whereas others may prefer complete silence. Observers may have questions; however, while the team is working, they should avoid talking unless they believe they are contributing information vital to patient care. Questions can often be posed during a break in the case or at the end of the procedure.

Scrubbed Individuals

During laparoscopic surgeries, the surgeon typically positions himself where it is most convenient to perform the operation. Thus, in cases in which laterality is involved, the surgeon usually stands on the side of the table opposite that of the pathology. In these cases, assistants and scrubbed individuals tend to stand on the same side of the patient table as the surgeon, allowing them to pass instruments to the surgeon and hold retracting instruments while the surgeon operates (Fig. 6.4). If an assistant is on the contralateral side

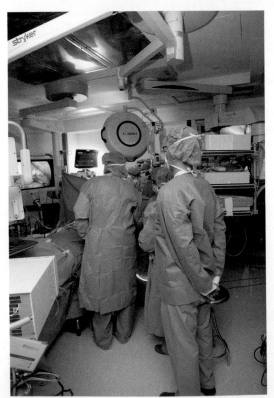

Fig. 6.1 Location in the OR of a nonscrubbed individual during a laparoscopic surgery

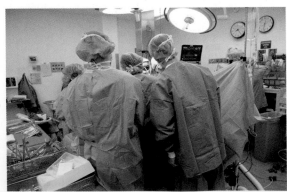

Fig. 6.2 Use of a standing stool to gain a better view of the operative field

of the table, she must be cognizant to stay out of the surgeon's line of sight of the primary video monitor.

During robotic surgeries, the surgeon and most observers remain unscrubbed. A surgical tech and first assistant will typically scrub for the procedure, and the first assistant will position himself at the patient bedside. As with laparoscopic surgeries, the laterality of the procedure usually dictates the side on which the assistant positions himself. During robotic procedures in which laterality is not applicable, such as in pelvic surgeries including robotic hysterectomy or prostatectomy, the position of the first assistant is dictated by surgeon preference and robotic

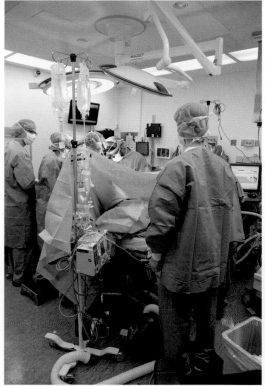

Fig. 6.3 Position of a nonscrubbed observer viewing a procedure from the anesthesia workspace

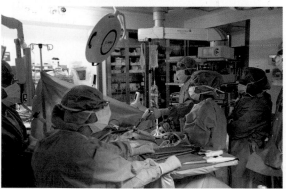

Fig. 6.4 Position of the surgeon and assistants on the left side of the table during a right laparoscopic surgery

trocar placement (Fig. 6.5). Other assistants may scrub for robotic surgeries as well, and their position may be on the same side or opposite that of the first assistant.

Open cases allow a high degree of variability in the position of the surgeon, assistants, and observers. By convention, the primary surgeon typically stands on the right side of the patient table during cases without laterality, although this may vary due to surgeon handedness and preference. When performing a procedure that involves laterality, the primary surgeon typically stands on the side of the table opposite the pathology during abdominal and pelvic procedures but may stand on the same side of the table as the surgical site during more accessible cases, such as orthopedic, skin, thoracic, vascular, or head and neck procedures. In many cases, the first assistant stands opposite the surgeon at the surgical site. Additional assistants and scrubbed observers may stand on either side of the table to allow them the best view of the surgical site. There needs to be minimal amount of interference between the scrub tech, surgeon, and first assistant. Additionally, assistants and observers at the table should avoid "stacking" between the scrub tech and the surgeon (Fig. 6.6).

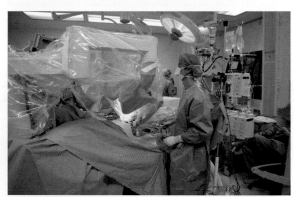

Fig. 6.5 Position of the first assistant at the patient bedside during a robotic-assisted laparoscopic surgery

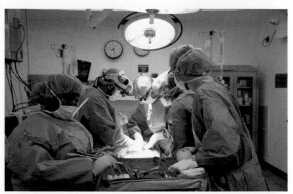

Fig. 6.6 Surgical team consisting of the primary surgeon and first assistant at the surgical site, the second assistant, observing medical student, and the scrub tech, allowing the scrub tech optimal access to the surgeon without stacking in between them

PASSING INSTRUMENTS

An important role of the scrub tech is to organize and pass instruments and supplies to the surgical team. Passing instruments in the correct way promotes efficient handling of devices and minimizes the risk of injury that many instruments and supplies may pose. Scrubbed assistants in the OR may act as an intermediary between the scrub tech and surgeon, and therefore it is important to understand how to hold and pass instruments.

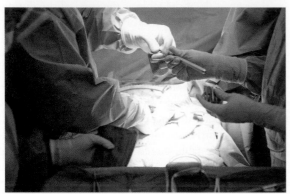

Fig. 6.7 Surgical instruments and supplies should always be passed over the surgical field.

In general, instruments should always be passed over the sterile surgical area. Passing instruments behind the back of a member of the surgical team or away from the field should be avoided, as it creates the potential for contamination, injury, and dropped or lost items (Fig. 6.7). The manner in which an instrument is passed depends on its intended use and should usually be presented in a manner that allows for immediate use. Instruments should usually be firmly placed in the palm of the dominant hand of the surgeon, as many times the surgeon cannot take her eye off the direct operative field. The presenter should release his grip just as he feels the surgeon has control. The surgeon usually calls out what instrument is needed next; however, experienced scrub techs who know the steps of the surgery can anticipate what is needed and automatically present the correct instrument.

Needle drivers should be passed to the surgeon with the needle loaded in the correct orientation for the surgeon to throw a suture. A right-handed surgeon usually requires that the needle be loaded differently than a left-handed surgeon. Additionally, the surgeon instructs the scrub tech if he will be throwing the needle in a forehand or backhand manner, and the needle should be loaded accordingly (Fig. 6.8). The surgeon requests the needle driver with an open palm, and the individual passing the needle driver places the handle (ring and

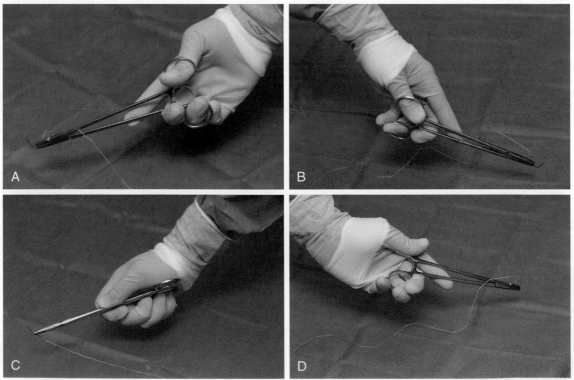

Fig. 6.8 Correct manner to load a needle onto a needle driver. A. Right-handed forehand-loaded needle driver. B. Left-handed forehand-loaded needle driver. C. Right-handed backhand-loaded needle driver. D. Left-handed backhand-loaded needle driver.

shank) of the driver in his hand (Fig. 6.9). The scrub tech should hold the driver at the mid portion of the shank, safely away from the exposed needle, as well as the handle where the surgeon will grasp the instrument. Passing an empty needle driver to the surgeon is similar to passing one that is already loaded with a needle; however, there is less concern for needlestick injury, and the individual passing the instrument may hold the driver near the jaws. In addition, before passing an empty needle driver or other ratcheted instrument, the ratchet should be closed. This locks the needle into position.

Passing a scissors is similar to passing a needle holder. As earlier, the surgeon extends an outstretched hand, and the scrub tech places the handle in his palm. Scissors should be closed before passing them to prevent injury. The individual passing the scissors may hold it by the closed blade or shank (Fig. 6.10). It is important to recognize the type of scissors being passed, as those with sharp and/or curved tips (e.g., Potts-Smith scissors) may increase the risk of injury if held incorrectly.

Retractors should be passed to the requesting individual so that the individual is able to grasp the handle (if present) and use the instrument immediately. To do this, the passing individual holds the retractor along the shank or blade of the instrument, then places the handle in the surgeon's palm (Fig. 6.11). Similarly, passing a grasping forceps, knife blade, or cautery device such as a Bovie electrocautery pen to a surgeon requires presenting it in a ready-to-use position. To receive these instruments, the surgeon extends his hand with his index finger and thumb in position to grasp the handle of the instrument (Fig. 6.12).

Returning instruments should be done in an organized fashion as well. When possible, surgeons should hand each instrument directly back to the scrub tech. However, this may not be possible when the surgeon is focused on the field, and therefore returned instruments should be placed on the operating table between the incision and the Mayo stand. Yet a surgeon may not always be able to do this and may place the instrument randomly on the table. Moreover, the scrub tech may be occupied securing the next tool the surgeon needs. As such, the operating table may become cluttered. This risks for instruments falling on the floor and becoming unsterile, and making an instrument difficult to find when it is needed. There is also personal danger to the team as they sort through a cluttered pile of instruments. The scrub tech works continuously to retrieve instruments and organize them on the Mayo stand and back table (Fig. 6.13). When not occupied directly with the incision, an assistant can help with gathering stray instruments. Additionally, redundant

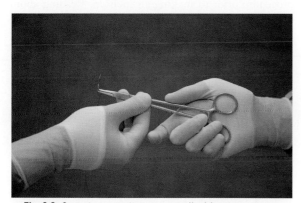

Fig. 6.9 Correct manner to pass a needle driver to a surgeon

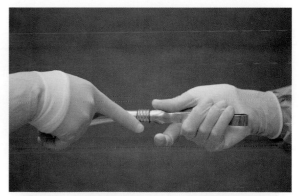

Fig. 6.11 Correct manner to pass a retractor to a surgeon

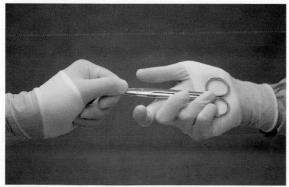

Fig. 6.10 Correct manner to pass a scissors to a surgeon

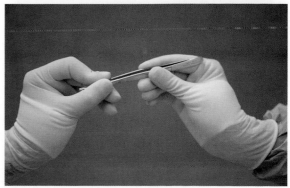

Fig. 6.12 Correct manner to pass a tissue-grasping forceps to a surgeon

suture material and other used supplies can clutter both the surgical field and sterile patient drapes. Suture material that still contains an unprotected needle may pose a risk to OR personnel and the patient, and should therefore be handed off the field for safe placement in a needle book as soon as its use is complete (Fig. 6.14). Suture material, clips, and other used supplies should be cleared from the surgical wound as they are used to prevent them from impeding working space.

When returning sharp instruments such as a knife or needle, the surgeon should actively call out the return to caution those at the table. These should be returned handle first under vision by the surgeon and the scrub tech.

EXPOSING THE FIELD

Exposure of the surgical field to allow a clean, clear, open working space is imperative in all surgical procedures. Open procedures necessitate constant attention to providing adequate exposure to the surgical wound by retracting, suctioning, and removing supplies and instruments from the immediate surgical field. During laparoscopic and robotic procedures, a working space is afforded by gas pneumoperitoneum; however, there are instances in which retraction may be beneficial.

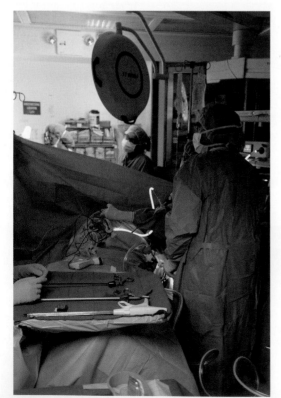

Fig. 6.13 Instruments and supplies should be organized in a manner to prevent them from cluttering the sterile field.

Identifying What Is Important

The most important first step in exposing the field is to allow the primary surgeon to clearly identify relevant surgical anatomy. A naive assistant can forget this principle and concentrate too much on her own vision. Sometimes the assistant can provide too much retraction, and in doing so may expose an irrelevant portion of the surgical field—or worse, inhibit the surgeon's performance by reducing working space. An experienced surgeon will place retractors in the correct position for an assistant to take over, and in time assistants will learn how to do so themselves.

In cases in which the surgical wound is relatively small, the entire field becomes relevant. Creation of an arteriovenous fistula for hemodialysis allows for a small wound in which all pertinent structures are confined to a small area. In contrast, an exploratory laparotomy for a small bowel obstruction exposes nearly the entire abdominal cavity. In this case, an adhesion that is typically confined to a small area necessitates a large surgical wound. Structures such as the pancreas, stomach, and great vessels are often encountered but are not the focus of the surgery. For this reason, it is important to identify what structures are important to avoid injuring them.

To identify which structures are important, it is crucial to understand the relevant anatomy of a surgical procedure prior to making an incision. Reading about the surgery and recognizing the relevant anatomy before entering the OR accomplishes this. Additionally, surgeons tend to concentrate their focus on the relevant anatomy of the case. By following the surgeon's movements and direction, one can often discern the important anatomical structures even without knowing what those structures may be.

Do No Harm

After determining the relevant anatomy of a procedure, it is important to understand how to help provide exposure to that anatomy. Retracting, suctioning, cutting suture, applying cautery, and other tasks may

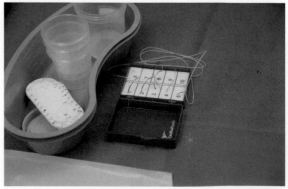

Fig. 6.14 Book of used needles

greatly help in exposing the field; however, they also have the potential to cause great harm. Forceful retraction has the potential to cause ischemia or even lacerate vital organs and vessels. Suctioning over recently placed liquid hemostatic agents may remove them. Past pointing with a scissors or electrocautery device and inadvertently lacerating other tissues can be devastating. It is for this reason that it is important to understand the task being performed and to know how to do it in an efficient and safe manner. Individuals should therefore be encouraged to ask for help or clarification when a task is unclear.

Retracting

Providing retraction in the field is central to exposing the surgical site of interest. Each tissue has both elasticity and memory, and intrinsically wants to return to its original orientation. As such, a continuous force is needed to move skin, fascia, tissue, and organs out of the way to allow manipulation. Self-retaining retractors allow a constant amount of force to be placed to expose a wound. These are most commonly used to hold skin or fascia aside. Longer, smoother blades are used to gently keep bowel and solid organs out of the way. By utilizing self-retaining retractors, assistant fatigue is prevented; a constant, steady, and predictable amount of retraction is provided; and assistants are free to help in other ways. Self-retaining retractors tend to be bulky, however, and may sometimes hinder surgeon movements. Additionally, they may be limited in the degree to which they can be manipulated (e.g., as with the Balfour retractor, which only provides a lateral spreading retraction), or it may be cumbersome and time consuming to change their position. Even more concerning is that the length and force of retraction may be great enough to cause tissue injury without recognition. As such, a folded, saline-moistened laparotomy pad may be used between a retractor and tissue to prevent tissue desiccation.

Handheld retractors are easily manipulated and less bulky than self-retaining retractors. Varying degrees of retractile force can be applied depending on the delicacy of the tissue being manipulated (Fig. 6.15). When using a handheld retractor, it is important to try to provide a steady amount of retractile force for the application for which it is being used. It is also important to hold the retractor steady and keep it at a constant angle and position on the tissue. Changing any of these variables may inhibit exposure of the surgical field or transiently obscure the field. Additionally, since the goal of using a retractor is to expose the field and allow the surgeon more working space, it is important to avoid getting in the way of the surgeon's movements while holding the retractor. When one is first learning, the assistant usually stays frozen and does not move for fear of interfering,

but with experience and understanding the steps of an operation, an assistant can actively move the retractor in a choreographed manner.

Manipulating a retractor in different ways may prevent assistant fatigue and strain, and minimize obstruction of the surgeon to working in the field. It is certainly acceptable to change the way a retractor is held during the course of retraction to provide better exposure and prevent

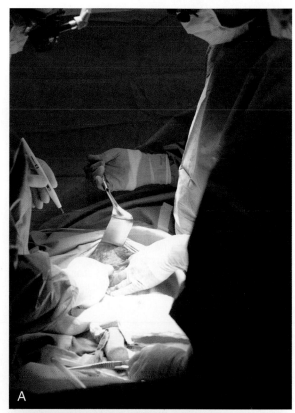

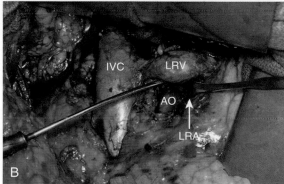

Fig. 6.15 Varying degrees of force may be utilized with handheld retractors. A. Forceful retraction of the abdominal wall to expose the abdominal cavity. B. Delicate retraction of the external iliac vein to expose the pelvic lymph nodes. IVC, inferior vena cava; LRV, left renal vein; AO, abdominal aorta; LRA, left renal artery. Used with permission from Karnes RJ, Blute ML. Surgery insight: management of renal cell carcinoma with associated inferior vena cava thrombus. *Nature Clinical Practice Urology.* 2008;5(6):329–339.

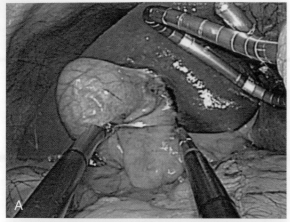

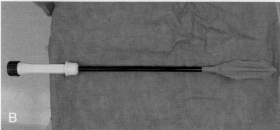

Fig. 6.16 Retraction during laparoscopic or robotic surgeries. A. Laparoscopic snake retractor. B. Laparoscopic paddle used for retraction during an intraabdominal laparoscopic surgery. Part A from Sung NS, Choi IS, Moon JI, Ra YM, Lee SE, Choi WJ. Four-channel single incision laparoscopic cholecystectomy using a snake retractor: comparison between 3- and 4-channel SILC 4-channel single incision cholecystectomy. *Annals of Surgical Treatment and Research.* 2014;87(2):81–86.

fatigue. When doing so, it is important to alert the team so that repositioning does not interfere with the operation.

Although a hand can be used as a retractor, when possible it is preferable to use instruments. Tools have a much lower profile and avoid potential inadvertent injury from operative instruments and needles. On the other hand, using a gloved hand to hold structures out of the surgical field provides tactile feedback to the assistant and prevents injury that may be caused by a metal instrument. Hand retraction, such as that which is employed to hold the bowel away from the operative site during intraabdominal surgeries, is typically delicate and not forceful. As tissues tend to be slippery, the use of a radiopaque towel, gauze, or lap pad may aid in traction without getting in the way of the surgical site.

Retraction of tissues during laparoscopic or robotic surgeries may also be necessary. Purpose-built laparoscopic paddles (Endo paddles) and snake retractors that expand when placed through a port site can be employed (Fig. 6.16).[1] These instruments are blunt and prevent injury to delicate tissues. After positioning a laparoscopic retractor, gentle traction is sufficient and helps in avoiding inadvertent injury.

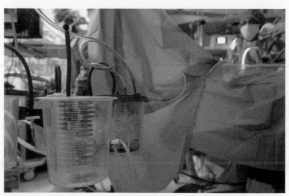

Fig. 6.17 Suction canister with tubing connected to wall suction and tubing running to the surgical field

KEEPING THE FIELD CLEAR

Suctioning fluids and removing debris from the wound are pivotal in keeping the surgical site visible. During open surgical procedures, an assistant often helps by suctioning and removing unneeded supplies, instruments, and debris from the field. Laparoscopic suction devices are utilized in robotic and laparoscopic surgeries. An astute assistant often greatly reduces the time spent in a procedure by ensuring that the surgeon has a clear field in which to work.

Suctioning

One of the simplest yet most helpful roles of an assistant during a surgical procedure is to clear the operative site of blood and other fluids. Additionally, there are many instances in which an irrigating fluid is poured into the wound to "wash" an area and subsequently removed by suction. A suction tip, such as a Yankauer, Poole, or Frazier suction tool is connected via tubing to centralized wall suction. In the suction line is a collection canister that holds the fluid for safe disposal and allows measurement of how much blood or fluid has been evacuated from the body.

Several important points should be remembered to be able to effectively clear the field using suction. First, there must be adequate negative pressure to be able to draw fluid from the surgical site. This negative pressure is provided by a wall suction unit connected to a tubing set that runs through the suction canister. From the suction canister, another tubing set runs to the surgical field and is connected to a suction tip. This latter suction tubing draws fluid into the canister where it is collected (Fig. 6.17). When a canister becomes full, negative pressure is released and suction from the surgical field ceases until a fresh canister is replaced. It is important to ensure that wall suction is functional prior to commencing a surgical case and to be vigilant about changing suction canisters before they become full.

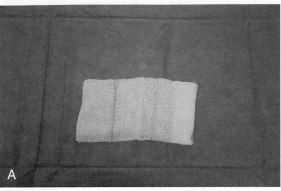
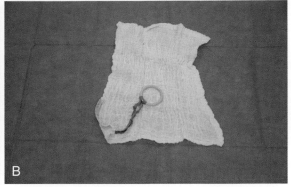

Fig. 6.18 Surgical gauze and pad. A. Surgical gauze with blue radiopaque marker. B. Laparotomy pad with blue radiopaque marker.

The second important point to consider is that debris, including suture material and tissue, often cannot pass through the suction tip. When the suction tip comes in contact with debris, it will be suctioned into the tip of the suction tool and clog it, preventing fluid from entering the suction tip. Blood clots may be deformable enough to pass through the suction tool, but they can clog the suction tip as well. All of the aforementioned debris may make its way through the suction tip and clog the tubing at any point in its course to the suction canister. It is therefore important to check the tip of the suction tool and tubing for debris when a loss of suction is encountered. Bulky debris, tissue, and large blood clots may be more efficiently removed from the surgical field using gauze pads or forceps. This also minimizes the risk of clogging the suction unit.

As with all facets of surgery, there is an art to suctioning. Practice is needed to become adept at this important aspect of surgery. The assistant should concentrate attention on where the surgeon is working. She should avoid placing the suction tool where it would obscure the surgeon's vision or interfere with instrument movement. In small spaces, the assistant must learn to dart in and out between a surgeon's manipulations. It is often tempting to clear blood and other fluids from surrounding areas of the surgical field where they may be collecting. In doing so, however, this may allow fluid to accumulate where the surgeon is working, if even for a brief time, and disrupt a surgeon's workflow. During a period of changing instruments, requesting a suture, or other break in the procedure, it may then be acceptable to clear fluids from the surrounding surgical field.

Gauze and Laparotomy Pads

Surgical gauze and laparotomy pads (Fig. 6.18) are also often used to clear the surgical field. They are constructed of absorbent cotton that rapidly wicks fluid. Both surgical gauze and laparotomy pads are equipped with radiopaque markers that are easily visible on x-ray (Fig. 6.19).[2] The material may be used to gently grasp

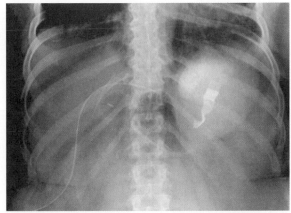

Fig. 6.19 Retained laparotomy pad in left upper quadrant, easily visible on plain x-ray. Reproduced with permission from Gibbs VC. Retained surgical items and minimally invasive surgery. *World Journal of Surgery*. 2011;35(7):1532–1539.

debris and remove it from the field. This is an especially effective method of clearing large blood clots that would otherwise clog suction tubing.

An important use of pads is to rapidly sop up accumulated blood and fluids. Forceful rubbing of a pad over tissue has the potential to create traction and abrasion injury. As such, the material should be dabbed over the area to be cleared. Additionally, pads can be used to pack and apply pressure to a bleeding area.

Pads and towels can also be used to retract structures away from the working site. They can be wadded up and packed to hold bowel back or unfurled to create a large surface area for which to retract tissue. When using these materials, a strict count with regard to the number of each that is opened onto the sterile field, and separately those placed inside the patient, is maintained. It is extremely important to ensure that no pieces of gauze or pads are left in the surgical site at the end of the procedure. Should an incorrect count of the number of either occur at the end of a procedure, an x-ray of the surgical site is required prior to surgical site closure.

HOLDING THINGS FOR THE SURGEON

Most open surgical procedures require at least one assistant, if not more, to help hold instruments and supplies for the primary surgeon during a procedure. This helps with retraction of tissues, placement of sutures, and visualization of the field.

Clamps

Providing retraction of tissues with specialized retractors, such as Richardson, Army-Navy, and Deaver retractors, allows significant mobilization of tissue. These retractors are typically large and move tissue in bulk. There are instances where more delicate structures need to be moved out of the way or presented to the surgeon for repair. Some clamps, including Kocher, Kelly, and Allis clamps, may be placed directly onto the tissue that needs to be retracted. Other clamps, such as Babcock clamps, may be placed around tubular structures to allow their retraction. For example, during repair of an inguinal hernia, retraction of the external oblique fascia with a handheld retractor would be cumbersome. Placing a small clamp on the fascia allows gentle, precise retraction needed for identification and closure. Clamps placed on bowel and blood vessels must be held gently to avoid tearing tissue. Only a minimum amount of force should be used to retract tissues with a clamp. As such, tissues are gently manipulated to present the area of interest to the surgeon for repair and can readily be moved to allow different views. It is important for an assistant to keep her hand and the clamp out of the line of sight of the surgeon to avoid impeding visualization of the working field. The surgeon will usually position the angle and clue the assistant on the degree of force desired; however, with experience, this will become intuitive for an assistant.

Sutures

Sutures come in a wide variety of materials, sizes, and lengths. Some suture is loaded onto a needle, whereas other sutures come "free," or without a needle. Surgeons often place sutures through tissue to allow apposition, as is common during fascial and skin closure of a wound. Sutures are also used to tie off structures, such as when a vessel is to be ligated. Although suture material, sizes, and how to suture are specifically discussed in Chapter 7, this section aims to describe how to most effectively aid a surgeon while he is suturing.

When a free suture is required, it can be delivered to the surgeon in one of two general ways. First, it can be handed to him without the aid of an instrument (Fig. 6.20). This allows the surgeon to manipulate the suture as he needs to tie off structures. Alternatively, it can be delivered to him on a passer (clamp) that has the suture loaded onto the end.

This allows the surgeon to place the suture where it would be more difficult to do so as a free suture, such as in deep spaces or those with minimal clearance. Many times, an assistant is asked to deliver the suture, loaded on a passer, to the surgeon so that he can grasp it with another instrument and perform a surgical tie (Fig. 6.21). The suture is loaded onto the tip of an instrument, typically either a curved or right-angle clamp, and the tip of the instrument is passed beneath the structure to be ligated. After the surgeon grasps the suture, the ratchet of the passer is released and the instrument is withdrawn. It is important to place a slight amount of tension on the back end of the suture during this process, allowing it to be drawn away from the passing instrument and more easily grasped.

When a running suture is being performed, it is important to have an assistant hold the suture and "follow" the surgeon as he throws it. To do this, the end of the suture that was most recently thrown by the surgeon is grasped by an assistant and retracted away from where the surgeon is to throw his subsequent sutures (Fig. 6.22). This allows the suture material to stay out of the surgeon's way, and provide tension to allow tissue apposition and prevent recently thrown sutures from sliding backward and loosening. When following, the assistant should not hold the suture too close to the needle, as this will limit the surgeon's ability to manipulate the needle. Additionally, the assistant should ensure that

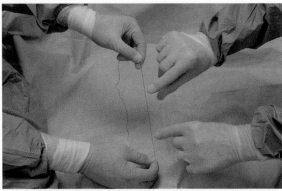

Fig. 6.20 Delivering suture to the surgeon as a free suture

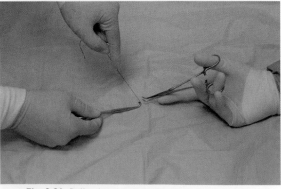

Fig. 6.21 Delivering suture to the surgeon on a passer

the suture does not get caught up on other instruments in the operative field.

It is important to understand how much tension to apply when following a surgeon's suture. Providing too little tension will allow laxity in the suture material and prevent good apposition of tissues, and can be detrimental in applications such as fascial closure. Alternatively, in some cases, providing too much tension can break suture material or cause buckling of the tissue and is unfavorable during applications such as performing a subcuticular skin closure.

Laparoscopes and Endoscopes

A particularly important job for an assistant during a laparoscopic surgery may be to hold the laparoscope. Laparoscopic surgeons typically operate using instruments in both hands and require someone else to hold the laparoscope for them. Although special camera holders are available to hold the laparoscope in place during surgery (Fig. 6.23), many surgeons favor an assistant holding the camera, as this allows it to be moved while the surgeon continues to operate.

Holding the laparoscope can be a difficult task for a new assistant in the OR (Fig. 6.24). It requires a steady hand to keep the scope from excessive movement. It also requires a rudimentary knowledge of the surgery being performed. Additionally, it requires the assistant

to be aware of the surgeon's movements and to know when to move the laparoscope to a different area of the field. In general, the laparoscope should be kept so that the surgeon's instruments are in the center of the view.

Just as a surgeon may require assistance in holding a laparoscope, during many endoscopic surgeries the surgeon may require an assistant to hold the endoscope, as well. While the assistant holds the endoscope, the surgeon passes instruments through it to perform the procedure (Fig. 6.25). This may be the case during multiple urologic surgeries, including cystoscopy and ureteroscopy, bronchoscopy, colonoscopy, and gastrointestinal endoscopic procedures. Although similar to holding a laparoscope, holding an endoscope requires a greater

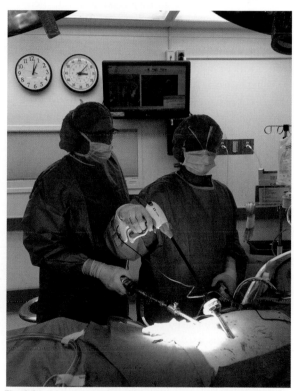
Fig. 6.24 Assistant holding a laparoscope in place during a laparoscopic surgery

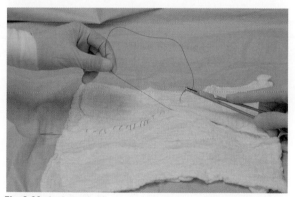
Fig. 6.22 Assistant holding suture material and following the surgeon as he performs a running suture

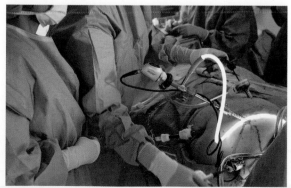
Fig. 6.23 Laparoscope holder with the laparoscope in place

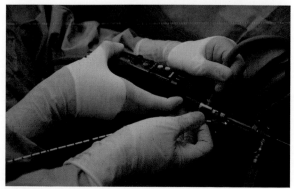
Fig. 6.25 Assistant holding a cystoscope (endoscope), allowing the surgeon to manipulate instruments through it during a cystoscopy

knowledge of the anatomy and surgical procedure being performed. Whereas an inexperienced assistant may be able to ascertain where he should be focusing the camera during a laparoscopic procedure, many endoscopic procedures require the camera to be directed to where it needs to be prior to other instruments being introduced. For this reason, holding an endoscope may be a bit more challenging for the inexperienced assistant in the OR.

CUTTING SUTURE

After a surgeon completes a surgical knot, redundant suture material is often cut and discarded. Cutting suture may seem to be an easy task; however, there are nuances. Should the needle be cut off before the surgeon begins to throw her knot? Should the suture be cut short, or should there be a tail left behind? What is the proper way to hold the suture scissors?

When cutting redundant suture material, only the tips of the scissors should be used (Fig. 6.26). This is especially relevant when cutting a suture within a surgical wound, as past pointing the tips of the scissors increases the chance that an injury to other structures may occur. It may be necessary to use a second hand to steady the scissors in some instances to prevent shaking of the tips of the scissors. When cutting suture material directly on the surgical knot, the tips of the scissors should be placed against the knot and turned at a 45-degree angle (Fig. 6.27). This prevents inadvertent cutting of the knot itself and allows a small amount of suture material to remain, preventing the knot from unraveling.

To correctly hold a suture scissors, the thumb and fourth finger are placed through the handle loops. The middle finger is used to support the lower edge of the instrument, whereas the index finger aids in supporting and directing the tips of the scissors (Fig. 6.28). Because most suture scissors are designed for use as right-handed

instruments, cutting is slightly different when performed with one's right hand compared to left hand. The natural position dictates that the thumb slightly pushes on the handle while the fourth finger slightly pulls. This allows the blades of the scissors to appose well and smoothly cut when used with the right hand (Fig. 6.29). This same motion, however, would cause

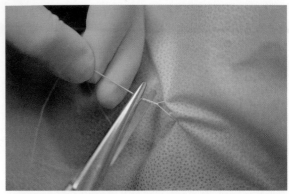

Fig. 6.27 Cutting suture material directly on the surgical knot requires the scissors to be turned at a 45-degree angle.

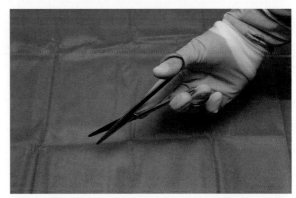

Fig. 6.28 Proper way to hold a suture scissors

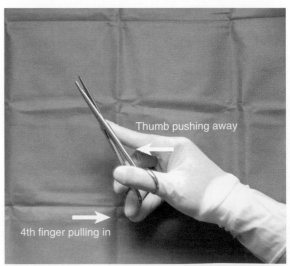

Thumb pushing away

4th finger pulling in

Fig. 6.29 Holding a suture scissors to cut with the right hand

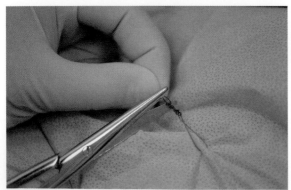

Fig. 6.26 When cutting suture material after tying a surgical knot, only the tips of the scissors should be used.

the blades of the scissors to separate when used with the left hand. For this reason, when cutting with one's left hand, the thumb must be used to slightly pull on its ring while the fourth finger pushes on its ring, allowing the blades of the instrument to come together (Fig. 6.30).

A continuous running suture requires the needle to be left attached after each throw of the suture (see Fig. 6.22).

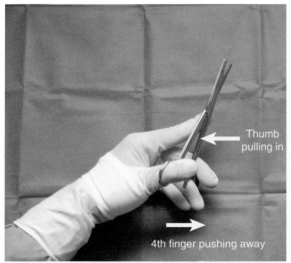

Fig. 6.30 Holding a suture scissors to cut with the left hand

Thumb pulling in

4th finger pushing away

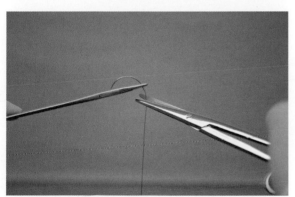

Fig. 6.31 Proper technique to cut a needle from the suture material, retaining as much suture as possible to throw a surgical knot

Interrupted sutures, however, may not require the needle to stay attached. If the surgeon plans to use the suture material for subsequent interrupted sutures, the needle should be left attached. If the remaining suture material will not be used again, cutting off the needle prior to the surgeon beginning to tie a knot can prevent needlestick injuries. In this case, the needle itself is grasped with a needle holder and the suture is cut at the base of the needle, allowing as much suture material as possible to remain to tie the surgical knot (Fig. 6.31).

One of the most difficult decisions that needs to be made when cutting redundant suture material is how much of a tail should be left on the knot (Fig. 6.32). If unsure, it is best to ask the surgeon how much of a tail should be left to avoid cutting the suture too short or too long. Monofilament suture material has a greater chance of unraveling and therefore requires a longer tail to remain on the knot. Too long of a tail can cause irritation and may erode through the closure site when close to the skin. However, braided sutures have a lesser chance of unraveling, and thus a short tail is sufficient.

APPLYING CAUTERY

Cautery is used during the course of a surgical procedure to provide an electrical-induced cut or to coagulate small blood vessels. The same instrument can often be used to perform both functions via different mechanisms. For example, using the Bovie monopolar electrocautery tool (Fig. 6.33), a surgical cut can be made by activating the "cut" function (typically a yellow button) and coagulation can be performed by activating the "coag" function (typically a blue button). It is important to note that instruments utilizing monopolar electricity will slightly disperse energy to surrounding tissues, whereas instruments that use bipolar energy will confine it to the area between the tips of the instrument.

When applying cautery, some important principles should be remembered. First, it is rare that a coagulating current should ever be used on exposed skin. By doing

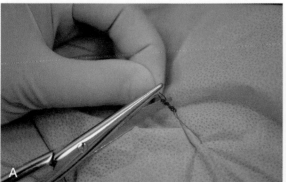
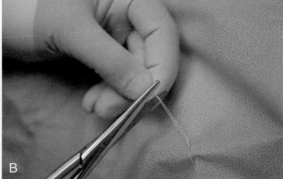

Fig. 6.32 Suture tail length after tying a surgical knot. A. Short tail length. B. Long tail length.

so, a burn injury occurs and a scar may develop. Alternatively, cutting current may be used with minimal risk of scar formation.

Oftentimes when applying cautery, a surgeon will expose the tissue to be cauterized. For example, a surgeon may utilize a right-angle or curved clamp to expose subcutaneous fat that is then divided with electrocautery. Unless otherwise instructed, exposed tissue should typically be cauterized in the middle of the exposed tissue, as opposed to nearer to one of the instrument tips (Fig. 6.34). Touching the cautery instrument to the metal instrument allows electricity to flow through the instrument, potentially injuring adjacent tissue. Additionally, when cauterizing tissue that has been exposed with a gloved finger, it is important to remember that the instrument becomes very hot. Therefore, the electrocautery tool should not be allowed to remain in one place for a prolonged period of time.

When cauterizing tissue over an area of bleeding, it is important to attempt to discern the bleeding vessel to the extent possible. If identified, a bleeding vessel can often be gently grasped with forceps and cautery applied to the forceps. This allows a current to run through the forceps and coagulate the bleeding vessel (Fig. 6.35). When directly coagulating an area of bleeding with the cautery tool, two general techniques may be used. A "touch buzz" technique is used when only a small bleeding vessel is suspected (Fig. 6.36). In this method, the cautery device is activated and the tip is briefly touched to the area of bleeding. However, in a "painting" technique, the cautery is activated and the tip of the instrument is run over a larger surface area of tissue. Painting tissue may be used when a more diffuse oozing of blood is suspected (Fig. 6.37).

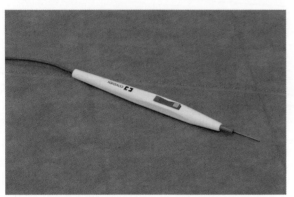

Fig. 6.33 Bovie electrocautery pen used to cauterize tissue

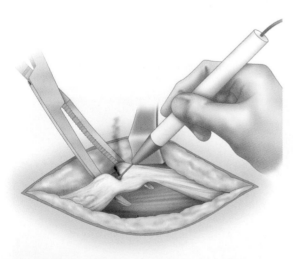

Fig. 6.34 Applying electrocautery to exposed tissue should typically be performed midway between the jaws of the instrument.

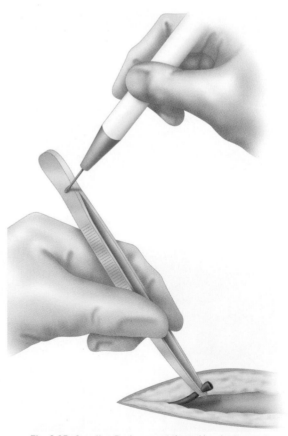

Fig. 6.35 Coupling Bovie current through an instrument

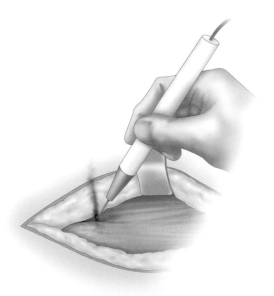

Fig. 6.36 Touch buzz technique used to coagulate small bleeding vessels

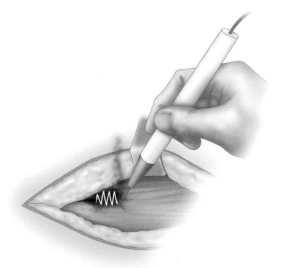

Fig. 6.37 Painting technique used to control diffuse oozing

REFERENCES

1. Sung NS, Choi IS, Moon JI, Ra YM, Lee SE, Choi WJ. Four-channel single incision laparoscopic cholecystectomy using a snake retractor: comparison between 3- and 4-channel SILC 4-channel single incision cholecystectomy. *Annals of Surgical Treatment and Research*. 2014;87(2):81–86.
2. Gibbs VC. Retained surgical items and minimally invasive surgery. *World Journal of Surgery*. 2011;35(7):1532–1539.

CHAPTER 7
SUTURES AND SUTURING

A fundamental aspect of surgery is reconstruction. This can be as pedestrian as skin closure or as complex as reattachment of a severed organ. Central to all reconstructive techniques is suturing various tissues back together. This is a practice that dates back centuries and likely was adapted from practices related to the use of needle and thread by tailors and garment makers. Modern suture material has evolved to be biocompatible and specialized for various applications. Sutures are used in most cases in the operating room (OR), in the emergency department to close lacerations, and in some cases on inpatient floors. This chapter reviews the basics of suturing and knot tying, along with an introduction to the different types of suture material.

SUTURE MATERIALS AND SIZES

Surgical sutures are available in a wide variety of materials, diameters, and tensile strength developed for specific situations. Suture material is available as either a free suture or attached to a needle. In addition to being available in a large variety of sizes, they may be absorbable or nonabsorbable, natural or synthetic, and braided or nonbraided. Absorbable sutures are dissolved by the body over time and used where natural ingrowth of tissue will provide sufficient strength over time. Nonabsorbable material is used when a longer period of healing is needed or when the suture will be used to mark the location of the surgical site for future surgeries. Natural sutures, including silk and chromic gut sutures, were widely used prior to the advent of synthetic sutures. However, these natural materials tend to create a greater inflammatory reaction in the body than synthetic sutures, which have more consistent performance and tend to be cheaper to produce. Braided sutures are easier to handle, as they do not have a memory, have less tendency to unravel or loosen in a surgical knot, and may require fewer ties to maintain the knot. Braided suture theoretically has a surface where blood cells can get trapped, however, and are therefore usually not used in low-flow venous repairs. Nonbraided (monofilament) sutures tend to produce less of an inflammatory response and slide through tissues more easily, as there is less friction from a single fiber passing through tissue. Needles come in various sizes and shapes, and with differing tips, to allow them to pass through a given tissue in an atraumatic fashion.

Suture Materials

Table 7.1 provides a concise overview of commonly used surgical sutures, as well as important characteristics of each suture material.

Absorbable Sutures

Absorbable sutures are classified as those sutures that are dissolved by the body over time. Different suture materials provide varying amounts of tensile strength and wound security, as well as inflammatory reaction. The actual time of dissolution and degree of inflammation is patient specific, and times mentioned are a rough guide, with actual times likely being a bit longer. Overall, these sutures tend to provoke a greater inflammatory response than nonabsorbable sutures. In general, absorbable sutures are not removed when used for skin closure and are valuable for internal use, as they allow sufficient tensile strength while dissolving over time, therefore eliminating foreign body material and a nidus for infection. The following suture materials are commonly used absorbable sutures.

Chromic gut (Fig. 7.1). This suture is made from the serosal lining of bovine or sheep intestine and processed with a chromium salt solution to reduce its absorption. Prior to the widespread production and use of synthetic sutures, chromic gut was one of the most commonly used natural suture materials. Although constructed as a monofilament, it does not slide through tissue as easily as most synthetic monofilament sutures. This property also allows it to hold securely in tissue and in surgical knots. Chromic sutures are useful when a rapidly dissolving suture is needed. It is therefore commonly used to close the skin edges of a wound in an interrupted fashion. Chromic gut induces one of the greatest inflammatory reactions of all suture material. It is typically absorbed within 90 days and retains its tensile strength for 3 to 4 weeks.

Table 7.1 Properties of Commonly Used Suture Materials

Suture	Origin	Braided or Monofilament	Available Sizes	Tensile Strength	Absorption Complete By
Absorbable sutures					
Chromic gut	Natural	Monofilament	7/0–3	21–28 days	90 days
Plain gut	Natural	Monofilament	6/0–0	7–10 days	70 days
Monocryl	Synthetic	Monofilament	6/0–1	1 week: 50–70% 2 weeks: 20–40%	91–119 days
Caprosyn	Synthetic	Monofilament	6/0–1	5 days: 60% 10 days: 20–30%	56 days
Biosyn	Synthetic	Monofilament	6/0–1	2 weeks: 75% 3 weeks: 40%	110 days
Vicryl	Synthetic	Monofilament Braided	M: 10/0–9/0 B: 8/0–3	2 weeks: 75% 3 weeks: 40–50%	56–70 days
PDS	Synthetic	Monofilament	7/0–2	2 weeks: 60–80% 6 weeks: 35–60%	182–238 days
Maxon	Synthetic	Monofilament	7/0–1	2 weeks: 75% 6 weeks: 25%	180 days
Nonabsorbable sutures					
Prolene	Synthetic	Monofilament	10/0–2	Indefinite	n/a
Mersilene	Synthetic	Monofilament Braided	M: 11/0–10/0 B: 6/0–1	Indefinite	n/a
Nylon	Synthetic	Monofilament	11/0–2	Gradual loss over time	n/a
Silk	Natural	Braided	7/0–2	Gradual loss over time	n/a
Stainless steel	Synthetic	Monofilament	5/0–7	Indefinite	n/a

M, monofilament; B, braided; n/a, not applicable.

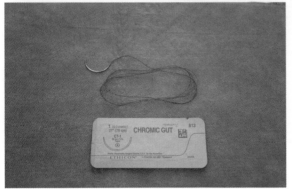

Fig. 7.1 Chromic gut suture. © Ethicon 2017. Reproduced with permission.

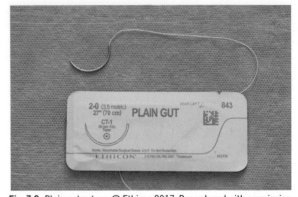

Fig. 7.2 Plain gut suture. © Ethicon 2017. Reproduced with permission.

Plain gut (Fig. 7.2). Similar to chromic gut, this suture is made from the serosal lining of bovine or sheep intestine but is not treated with a chromium salt solution. This increases the absorbability of the suture material in tissue and decreases its period of tensile strength to 7 to 10 days. Plain gut suture material is used in similar applications as chromic gut suture, although its use has been restricted to applications in which the necessary period of tensile strength is low.

Poliglecaprone 25 (Monocryl) (Fig. 7.3). This suture material is commonly used for subcuticular skin suturing. It is a monofilament suture that easily passes through tissue and creates a minimal tissue

reaction. Monocryl provides acceptable tensile strength to keep the edges of a wound together for approximately 14 days.

Biosyn (Fig. 7.4). Similar to Monocryl, this suture material is often used for subcuticular skin suturing. It provides slightly greater tensile strength than Monocryl sutures but is completely absorbed within the same time frame.

Caprosyn (Fig. 7.5). This suture material handles similarly to Monocryl and Biosyn in that it is easily passed through tissue and provides an acceptable tensile strength to provide skin closure during the initial healing process. However, it is completely

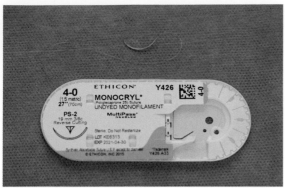

Fig. 7.3 Monocryl suture. © Ethicon 2017. Used with permission.

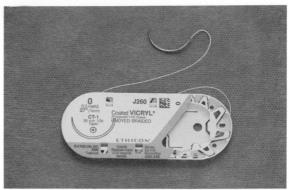

Fig. 7.6 Vicryl suture. © Ethicon 2017. Used with permission.

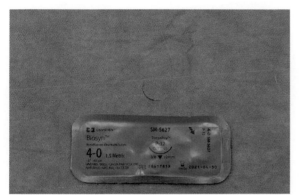

Fig. 7.4 Biosyn suture

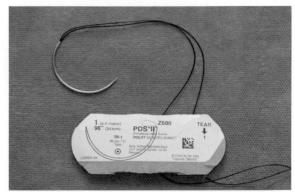

Fig. 7.7 PDS suture. © Ethicon 2017. Used with permission.

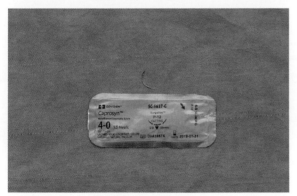

Fig. 7.5 Caprosyn suture

absorbed in about half the time of Monocryl and Biosyn, and theoretically decreases the risk of infection and inflammation to a greater degree than either of the suture materials mentioned previously. It provides a slightly reduced amount of tensile strength, though, with secure wound approximation for 10 days.

Polyglactin 910 (Vicryl) (Fig. 7.6). Vicryl suture material is commonly used for reapproximating subcutaneous tissue such as fat, muscle, and fascia. It is also commonly used for the ligation of small blood vessels, creation of surgical anastomoses, and

general-purpose suturing applications. It is a braided suture that easily passes through tissue and holds well in surgical knots. It provides excellent wound security with 40 to 50% tensile strength remaining at 3 weeks, although is completely absorbed by 70 days, minimizing the risk of long-term foreign body–related infection.

Polydioxanone (PDS) (Fig. 7.7). This monofilament suture is easily passed through tissue, provides excellent wound security for an extended period of time, and is completely absorbed by approximately 238 days. This makes PDS an optimal suture material for applications in which an extended period of wound support is desired in combination with a suture material that will still be absorbed. It is therefore commonly used for closure of the abdominal fascia and is available as a double-stranded looped suture material for this purpose.

Polyglyconate (Maxon) (Fig. 7.8). This suture material handles similarly to PDS and is available for similar applications. Like PDS, it is available in a double-stranded looped form for a running abdominal fascia closure. It provides extended wound support for up to 6 weeks but is absorbed slightly faster than PDS at 180 days.

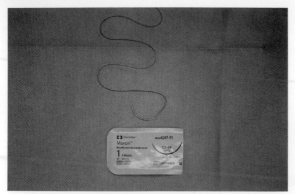

Fig. 7.8 Maxon suture

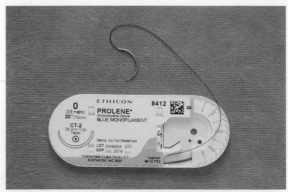

Fig. 7.9 Prolene suture. © Ethicon 2017. Reproduced with permission.

Nonabsorbable sutures

Nonabsorbable suture material is meant to be permanent and is not degraded over time by the body. It is often used when continued tensile strength over time is necessary, such as in cardiovascular surgical procedures. Since nonabsorbable sutures also tend to create less of an inflammatory reaction than absorbable sutures, they are useful for applications in which scar formation is undesirable, such as for skin closure on the head and neck. The following suture types are commonly used nonabsorbable sutures.

Polypropylene (Prolene) (Fig. 7.9). This monofilament suture is easily passed through tissue and causes minimal trauma as it does so. It provides excellent holding power and does not lose tensile strength over time. This makes it ideal for use in high-stress environments, such as the cardiovascular system, in which repeated pulsations and movements require extended wound support. Because of its high plasticity and smooth surface, it can easily unravel and thus extra surgical knot throws are required to maintain adequate knot strength.

Polyester (Mersilene) (Fig. 7.10). This suture material is a braided, nonabsorbable suture with excellent tensile strength. As opposed to Prolene, it maintains better knot hold because of its braided construction. It is useful in high-stress environments, such as large vessel vascular suturing. Because it is braided and may allow for additional bacterial adherence, it should not be used when infection is present. Additionally, platelet adherence is also possible, making it undesirable when repairing venous structures.

Polyamide; Nylon (Fig. 7.11). This is a monofilament suture that, although not absorbed, loses tensile strength over time. It is a very smooth suture with high plasticity that creates a minimal inflammatory reaction. It is commonly used to suture drains to the skin, as it is easily handled and creates minimal pain when removed.

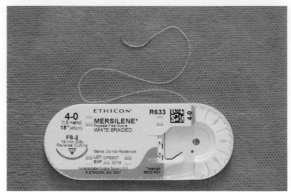

Fig. 7.10 Mersilene suture. © Ethicon 2017. Reproduced with permission.

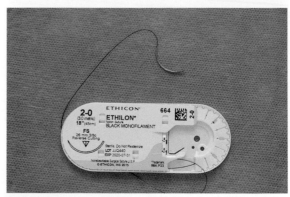

Fig. 7.11 Nylon suture. © Ethicon 2017. Reproduced with permission.

Silk (Fig. 7.12). This braided suture material is highly effective at ligating large vessels because of its ease of handling, long duration of tensile strength, and minimal unraveling in surgical knots. Although it is degraded slowly over time, it is not absorbed and is therefore useful in cases in which wound reentry and ease of locating the suture is anticipated. Because it is braided and does not become absorbed, it is slightly more prone to infection.

Stainless steel (Fig. 7.13). This monofilament suture material is utilized when significant tensile strength is needed. It is commonly used for

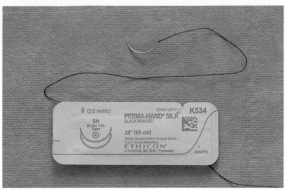

Fig. 7.12 Silk suture. © Ethicon 2017. Reproduced with permission.

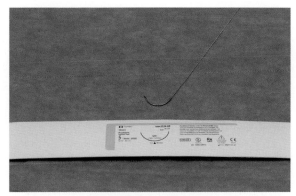

Fig. 7.13 Stainless steel suture

Table 7.2 Suture Sizes and Their Corresponding Diameters

Suture Size	Synthetic Absorbable Suture Minimum Diameter (mm)	Nonabsorbable Suture Minimum Diameter (mm)
10-0	0.02	0.02
9-0	0.03	0.03
8-0	0.04	0.04
7-0	0.05	0.05
6-0	0.07	0.07
5-0	0.10	0.10
4-0	0.15	0.15
3-0	0.20	0.20
2-0	0.30	0.30
0	0.35	0.35
1	0.40	0.40
2	0.50	0.50
3	0.60	0.60
4	0.60	0.60
5	0.70	0.70
6		0.80
7		0.90

Modified from http://www.pharmacopeia.cn/v29240/usp29nf24s0_m80190.html and http://www.pharmacopeia.cn/v29240/usp29nf24s0_m80200.html

sternal closure after cardiac surgical procedures and may be used in some orthopedic cases as well. It provides excellent knot security while creating relatively low tissue reactivity.

Suture Sizes

Suture size is defined by a number system and was originally manufactured in sizes ranging from #1 to #6, with successively increasing numbers designating thicker suture material. A #1 surgical gut suture has a minimum diameter of 0.4 mm. Each increase in number increases the diameter by 0.1 mm. With improvements in manufacturing techniques, smaller suture sizes were developed. They were given the designation of #00 (2-0 or 2/0, pronounced "two-oh"), #000 (3-0 or 3/0, pronounced "three-oh"), and so on, with each smaller diameter adding an additional zero. Note, however, that there is not a linear decrease in diameter as suture size decreases (Table 7.2). Additionally, there can be slight variability in diameter of a given size among suture classes (e.g., synthetic vs. natural suture material). Suture sizes range from #11/0 monofilament material used for the smallest microsurgical ophthalmic procedures to as large as #7 used for sternal wound closure. In general, the smallest suture material should be chosen that is still strong enough to approximate tissue. This

minimizes tissue reaction and inflammation while still providing adequate tensile strength.

Several common suture sizes are used for standard suturing applications, although these are modifiable based on patient and tissue characteristics, as well as surgeon preference. For example, subcuticular skin suturing in adults is often performed with a #4/0 size Monocryl, Caprosyn, or Biosyn suture. Subcutaneous fat closure is often performed with a #3/0 or #2/0 absorbable suture material such as Vicryl or chromic gut. Abdominal fascial closure typically dictates that a thicker suture material be used. When performing an interrupted figure-of-eight closure, common suture sizes include #0 and #1, typically with a Vicryl, Prolene, or PDS suture material. When performing a running fascial closure, as is often done with larger laparotomy wounds, a #0 or #1 looped PDS or looped Maxon suture may be used. Intricate vascular suturing and anastomoses are often performed with Prolene suture, with the size of the suture depending on the caliber of the vessel.

NEEDLE TYPES AND SIZES

A variety of needle types are available for different suturing applications. They can be straight or curved, tapered or blunt, and free or swaged (attached to suture material), and are available in several different thicknesses and arc diameters. Most needles are disposable, including all swaged needles, although some free needles are reusable after sterilization. They are usually constructed of surgical stainless steel.

Needle Shape

Surgical needles can be either straight or curved, although straight needles have limited use in the OR (Fig. 7.14). Straight needles can be used to suture skin edges closed, or in some cases to secure drains to the skin. They almost always contain a cutting point.

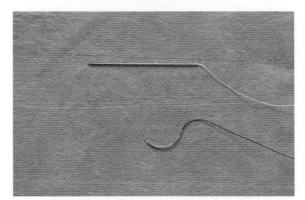

Fig. 7.14 Straight and curved surgical needles

Straight needles are usually handheld, as opposed to curved needles that require the use of a needle driver.

Curved needles are classified by the diameter of their arc. Commonly used curved needles include those that contain 1/4, 3/8, 1/2, and 5/8 circular arcs (Fig. 7.15). The degree of curvature of a needle may help with throwing sutures in different situations. For example, in deep surgical wounds in which instrument maneuverability is difficult, a needle with a greater curvature may help in throwing a suture. This is opposed to superficial, easily accessed tissue, in which a needle with less of a curvature may be easier to throw.

Needle Point

A variety of needle tip designs are available for different suturing applications. The most commonly used types include tapered needles, blunt needles, cutting needles, and reverse cutting needles.

Taper (Fig. 7.16). This needle tip, as its name suggests, gradually tapers down from the body to a sharp tip. The needle shaft itself is round throughout. This design allows tapered needles to stretch tissue as opposed to cutting it, allowing for the tissue to retract around the suture material after the needle has been passed through it, rendering the hole through which it passed as small as possible. This type of needlepoint is therefore relatively atraumatic to tissue. Tapered needles are the most commonly used

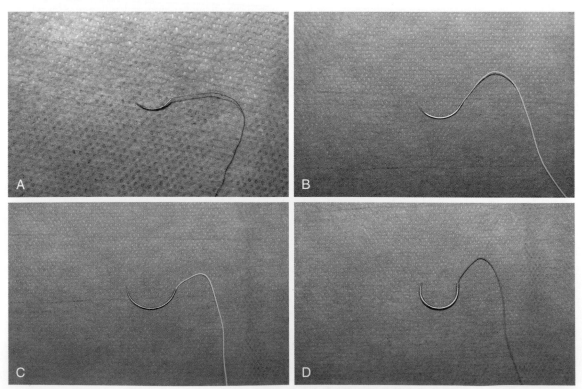

Fig. 7.15 Curved surgical needles. A. ¼ circle. B. 3/8 circle. C. ½ circle. D. 5/8 circle.

needles and have applications in all tissue types, except dense tissue such as skin. Common tapered needle designations include UR, CT, RB, and SH needle types. UR needles (UR-4, UR-5, and UR-6) are 5/8 circle taper point needles. By convention, increasing numbers generally denote smaller needle sizes within a given needle class. CT (CT, CT-1, CT-2, CT-3), RB (RB-1, RB-2, RB-3), and SH (SH, SH-1, SH-2) needles are all 1/2 circle taper point needles. CT needles are greater in diameter and thickness than SH needles, which are greater in diameter and thickness than delicate RB needles.

Blunt (Fig. 7.17). This needle contains a round shaft that slightly tapers down to a blunt point at the tip of the needle. It therefore requires a greater amount of force to be able to penetrate tissue than taper point needles. The use of blunt needles reduces needlestick injuries to OR personnel and the patient, although it makes driving these needles through tough tissue more difficult than with tapered needles. They are useful for applications that do not require suturing tough tissue, such as when reapproximating subcutaneous fat. BP (BP, BP-1, BP-2) needles are 1/2 circle blunt point needles often used for this purpose and have a large diameter. Alternatively, CTB (CTB, CTB-1, CTB-2) needles are also 1/2 circle blunt point needles, but have a smaller diameter.

Cutting (Fig. 7.18). This needle contains three cutting surfaces at the tip of the needle. The body of the needle is triangular and tapers down to a sharp point, with the cutting edge at the tip. As such, the cutting point lacerates tissue, causing more trauma than tapered needles. The cutting point itself, which is on the concave, inner surface of the needle, cuts in the direction of the needle pull through tissue. It is useful for suturing through dense or scarred tissue and is the most commonly used needle for skin closure. V-designated needles represent cutting needles and are available in either 3/8 circle (V-26, V-4) or 1/2 circle (V-5, V-7, V-34, V-37, V-40, V-56) diameters.

Reverse cutting (Fig. 7.19). This needle is similar to the cutting needle, except it contains the cutting edge on the convex, outer edge of the needle. This effectively places the cutting edge away from the direction of needle pull, preventing accidental cutting through tissue. This does, however, allow the needle to create larger holes than conventional cutting needles. This needle type is commonly employed in the placement of retention sutures. One such example is the CP needle type (CP, CP-1, CP-2), which represents a 1/2 circle reverse cutting needle.

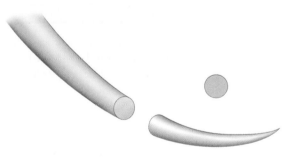

Fig. 7.16 Taper needle

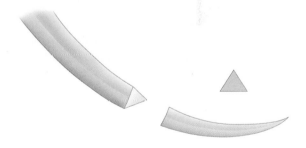

Fig. 7.18 Cutting needle

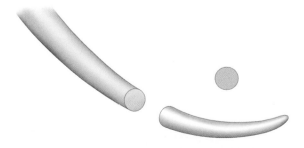

Fig. 7.17 Blunt needle

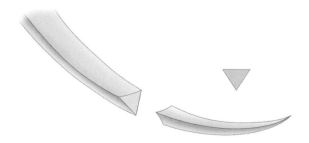

Fig. 7.19 Reverse cutting needle

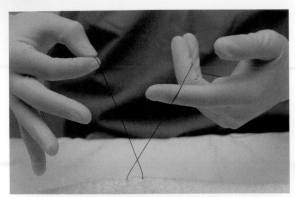

Fig. 7.20 Free compared to swaged surgical needle

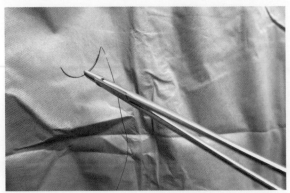

Fig. 7.21 Needle positioned in a needle holder at the midpoint of its curve

Free Versus Swaged Needles

Free needles are those that require a suture to be threaded through the eyelet at the end of the needle. This is opposed to the more common swaged needles that come preloaded with suture material (Fig. 7.20). Free needles are usually thicker than swaged needles, owing to the requirement for a large enough eyelet to thread suture material. Free needles are useful when the direction in which a suture was thrown needs to be reversed. This is the case when a swaged needle is thrown through tissue in one direction and the second throw of the suture requires that the opposite, needleless end of the suture be thrown through tissue as well. In this case, placing a free needle on the tail of the suture allows it to be thrown through tissue. Although some sutures have a double-armed construction for this purpose (such that there is a needle at both ends), most are single armed.

Swaged needles are available with both permanently attached suture materials, requiring the needle to be cut from the suture, and "pop-off" needles. The latter needles are released from the suture material with a gentle tug after throwing a suture. The advantage of this is that multiple single sutures can be thrown without stopping to cut the needle from the suture.

Needle Thickness and Circular Diameter

Needle thickness and circular diameter are primarily dependent on the caliber of suture material to which the needle is attached. This allows the needle to create a hole of adequate size to permit the suture material to pass through it, without making the defect in the tissue too large. An appropriate circular diameter of a needle allows the needle to easily be handled, without being excessively large or too small.

Smaller suture material is often used for suturing more delicate tissue, and larger suture material is used for more robust, thick tissue requiring greater tensile strength. As such, smaller needles easily pass through delicate tissue, whereas larger needles are better equipped to penetrate more dense tissue. However, there is a slight variation in needle

thickness that may be chosen for a given suture size. These are described as fine, medium, or heavy needles. Medium needle thickness is the most commonly used needle thickness. These needles are used for most surgical suturing. Fine needles, alternatively, are often employed when suturing delicate tissue, such as the bowel. Fine needles easily penetrate delicate tissue without creating an excessively large defect in the tissue. Heavy needles, also known as hernia needles, are used for penetrating dense, scarred tissue. They are useful when a medium-thickness needle would have difficulty passing through tissue, creating a concern for needle bending or breakage. When throwing a suture, care must be taken not to exert too much force, as this could lead to bending or breaking of the needle.

HOW TO THROW A SUTURE

Video 7.1 demonstrates the various techniques of how to throw a suture. A needle needs to be matched to an appropriate needle driver. Small, delicate needles need smaller drivers to prevent damaging the needle. Similarly, large needles require heavy drivers to grasp and push needles through tissue. In general, a needle should sit squarely in a needle holder, directly at the midpoint of its curve (Fig. 7.21). The needle itself is flat at this portion and therefore sits securely in the needle driver. This allows pronation of the hand to best control the tip. If the needle is positioned in the driver too close to the tip of the needle, the rounded body will cause the needle to move as it is being passed, and force can cause the needle to bend or break. Sometimes there are instances in which a surgeon will need to "choke up" on the needle and position it further toward the suture, therefore obtaining a better angle to gather tissue over the suture (Fig. 7.22). Additionally, when entering tissue, it is optimal to enter at a 90-degree angle to the tissue. This minimizes the size of the hole created by the needle and takes the most advantage of the tip shape to minimize the force of penetration. In addition, when

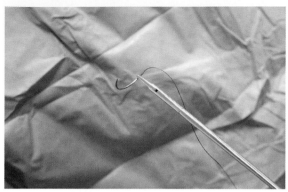

Fig. 7.22 "Choking up" on a needle

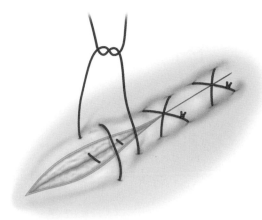

Fig. 7.24 Figure-of-eight suture

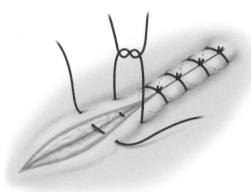

Fig. 7.23 Interrupted suture

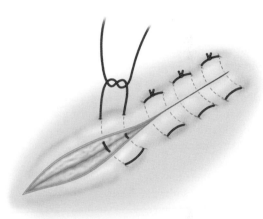

Fig. 7.25 Horizontal mattress suture

gathering tissue, one generally wants to incorporate an equal amount from each side of an incision.

Interrupted suture (Fig. 7.23). The simple interrupted suturing technique is one of the most commonly used methods of repairing tissue. It is often employed to close skin, reconstruct blood vessels, or reapproximate muscle and subcutaneous fat. With this suturing technique, the needle enters the tissue on the outside of one wound edge and is driven through to the inside of that wound edge. Regrasping the needle, it then crosses the wound and enters the opposite wound edge on the inside of the wound, penetrating the tissue and reemerging on the outside of the wound. A surgical knot is then tied to bring the two ends of the suture material together, thereby bringing the edges of the wound together.

A commonly used variation of the simple interrupted suture is the figure-of-eight suture (Fig. 7.24). In the same way a simple interrupted suture is thrown, the needle is driven through each side of the wound so that the ends of the suture are on the outside of the wound. Without tying a surgical knot, a second throw of the needle is performed

in the same direction as the first, bringing the needle out of the opposite side of the wound from the suture tail. A surgical knot is then tied. This method of wound closure effectively permits two interrupted sutures to be thrown per surgical knot, increasing the strength of the suture and decreasing tension by spreading the force over a wider area of tissue. This theoretically can decrease suture tearing through tissue.

Horizontal mattress suture (Fig. 7.25). This suturing technique is often used when delicate or poor-quality tissue must be reapproximated. It is useful in that it distributes and minimizes the tension placed on tissue while providing good tissue eversion. In the same manner a simple interrupted suture is thrown, the needle enters the wound edge on the outside of the wound and is driven to the inside of the tissue. The needle is then regrasped and driven through the inside of the opposite wound edge so that it reemerges on the outside

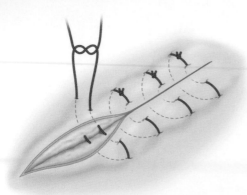

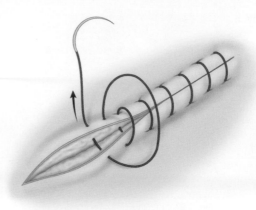

Fig. 7.26 Vertical mattress suture

Fig. 7.27 Running suture

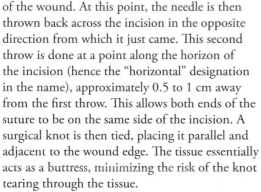

of the wound. At this point, the needle is then thrown back across the incision in the opposite direction from which it just came. This second throw is done at a point along the horizon of the incision (hence the "horizontal" designation in the name), approximately 0.5 to 1 cm away from the first throw. This allows both ends of the suture to be on the same side of the incision. A surgical knot is then tied, placing it parallel and adjacent to the wound edge. The tissue essentially acts as a buttress, minimizing the risk of the knot tearing through the tissue.

Vertical mattress suture (Fig. 7.26). This suturing technique is similar to the horizontal mattress suturing technique and is extremely effective at decreasing the dead space of a wound and enhancing wound edge eversion. Like the horizontal mattress suture, it decreases the tension placed on fragile tissue. Because it everts tissue, when used on the skin the suture may dig in and create stitch mark scars.

To throw a vertical mattress suture, a "far-far-near-near" or "near-near-far-far" technique of placing sutures is utilized. To perform the far-far-near-near technique, the needle is first driven through the outside of one edge of a wound at a distance that is "far" from the wound edge (in most skin closure applications, this is a distance of approximately 1 cm from the edge of the wound). The needle emerges on the inside of the wound and is then driven in an inside-out manner at a far distance through the opposite side of the wound. From the same side of the wound that the needle just emerged, the needle is thrown back across the wound at a "near" distance (approximately 0.5 cm or less from the wound edge). The two ends of the suture are then tied on the same side of the wound.

Running suture (Fig. 7.27). A running suture is performed as a faster alternative to the various interrupted suturing techniques. In this technique, a

simple interrupted suture is placed across one end of an incision and a surgical knot is tied. Instead of cutting the long end of the suture, however, it remains attached and is used to continue to throw sutures across the wound successively along the length of the incision. After reaching the opposite side of the incision, a surgical knot is thrown to complete the suture. It is important to maintain even spacing between suture throws when utilizing a running suture technique.

Running sutures, although faster than interrupted suturing techniques, may not be as secure as interrupted sutures. They may allow for gaps in the wound or, alternatively, bunching of wound edges. Unraveling of one knot or a break in the suture at any point along the incision allows the entire wound to open. This is as opposed to an interrupted suturing technique, in which breaking of one suture only allows the wound to open at that spot. For this reason, running sutures are only used to close skin where a great amount of tensile strength is not necessary and the skin has favorable healing characteristics. Alternatively, running sutures are often used to close the abdominal fascia. A running suture technique here is effective, as it distributes tension along the length of the fascial incision.

Subcuticular suture (Fig. 7.28). This running suturing technique is used only to reapproximate the edges of a skin incision. The technique is meant to allow apposition of the skin edges without visible suture and without the need for suture removal. Thus, a dissolvable suture such as Monocryl, Biosyn, or Caprosyn is often chosen. To initiate a subcuticular suture, a knot is first secured at one end of the wound. This is typically thrown through the subcutaneous tissue below the skin edge. The needle then enters the apex of the incision parallel to the skin surface at the dermal-epidermal junction. The needle passes through the dermal skin layer by following the curve of

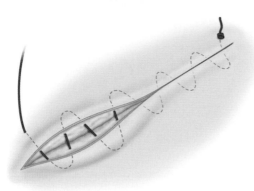

Fig. 7.28 Subcuticular suture

the needle. The next throw of the suture begins on the opposite side of the wound, at a point in line with the exit site of the previous needle throw. This allows the edges of the wound to line up as they were prior to an incision being made. Successive throws of the needle are performed on alternating sides of the incision until reaching the opposite end of the wound. After performing a surgical tie, the knot is buried by driving the needle from the inside of the apex of the incision to the outside of the wound. The suture is cut at the skin surface. Burying the knot in this manner helps to minimize patient discomfort from the knot.

KNOT TYING

Tying surgical knots is a key component of suturing, and proper technique is imperative to ensure a good outcome. In the case of a running suture, the surgical knot initiates and terminates the suturing process. Interrupted sutures essentially are surgical knots that hold two tissues together.

Monofilament suture tends to have a memory and may unravel if there are insufficient throws in the knot. As such, generally six separate throws are made to secure this material, and a relatively long tail is kept to prevent it from unraveling. Braided suture material usually requires a minimum of three throws to form a knot, and the tail can be relatively shorter. Tissue that is under tension or would result in significant consequences should a surgical knot break or unravel may dictate that a greater number of surgical knots be performed. An example of this is in closing the abdominal fascial layer. Conversely, when approximating tissue under minimal tension, a large surgical knot could cause irritation and discomfort (e.g., skin, subcutaneous fat, muscle), and

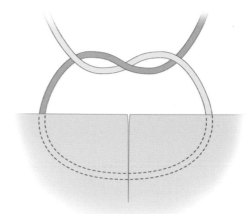

A

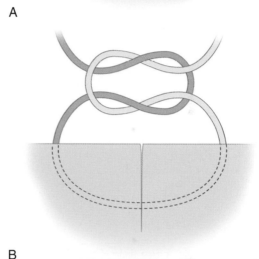

B

Fig. 7.29 Square knot. A. Initial throw of a square knot. B. Subsequent throws of a square knot.

fewer throws may be performed. Video 7.2 demonstrates the various techniques to tie a surgical knot.

Square Knot

Square knots are the standard for surgical knot tying. Performed correctly, they allow the knot to securely hold a suture in place without slippage. Square knots consist of alternating directions of suture throws to secure the knot in place. They can be performed with two-handed, one-handed, and instrument tying techniques.

One complete square knot consists of both a forehand and a backhand throw of the suture. With the initial throw, the suture material effectively lies such as that depicted in Fig. 7.29A before being drawn taut. Typically, multiple continuously alternating throws are performed to add security to a surgical knot (Fig. 7.29B). Although additional throws do provide assurance that the knot will hold well and not unravel, it also increases the bulkiness of the knot.

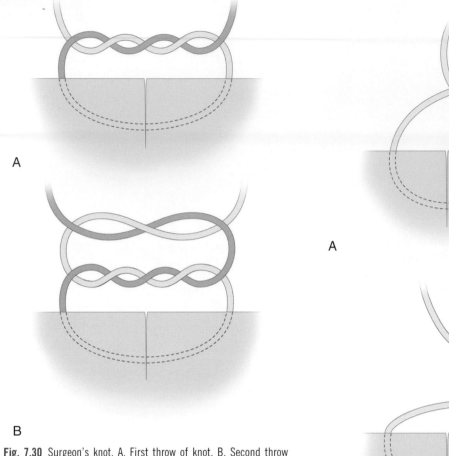

A

B

Fig. 7.30 Surgeon's knot. A. First throw of knot. B. Second throw of knot.

Surgeon's Knot

A surgeon's knot is a variation of the standard square knot that incorporates an extra twist of the suture material when performing the first throw. The suture material lies such as that depicted in Fig. 7.30 before being drawn taut. Successive throws of the suture are performed exactly as one would throw a square knot. The additional twist of the suture material provides more friction and prevents loosening of the suture prior to the second throw being performed. This knot allows tension to remain on the suture material and keep wound edges together until the second throw of the suture secures the knot in place. This is helpful when there is tension that would pull the tissues apart.

Slip Knot

A slip knot is performed similarly to a square knot. As opposed to square knots, which can be tied with two-handed, one-handed, and instrument tying techniques, slip knots are usually performed using a two-handed technique. Slip knots allow one arm of the suture material to be used as a rail to slide the other arm of the suture over it. This requires that tension be maintained on the

A

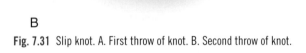

B

Fig. 7.31 Slip knot. A. First throw of knot. B. Second throw of knot.

arm of the suture that was used as the rail (Fig. 7.31). As opposed to a standard square knot, the second throw of the suture is usually performed in the same direction as the first. This allows for knot tightening without locking the suture material in place, thus minimizing air knots (a knot that is not firmly against tissue, allowing space for tissue to separate) from being thrown.

Two-Handed Knots

Two-handed surgical ties (Fig. 7.32) are the most reliable and easiest surgical knots to perform. Surgeons should become comfortable with throwing two-handed surgical knots while using each hand as the dominant hand.

In performing a two-handed surgical tie, both an "overhand" and "backhand" throw must be performed

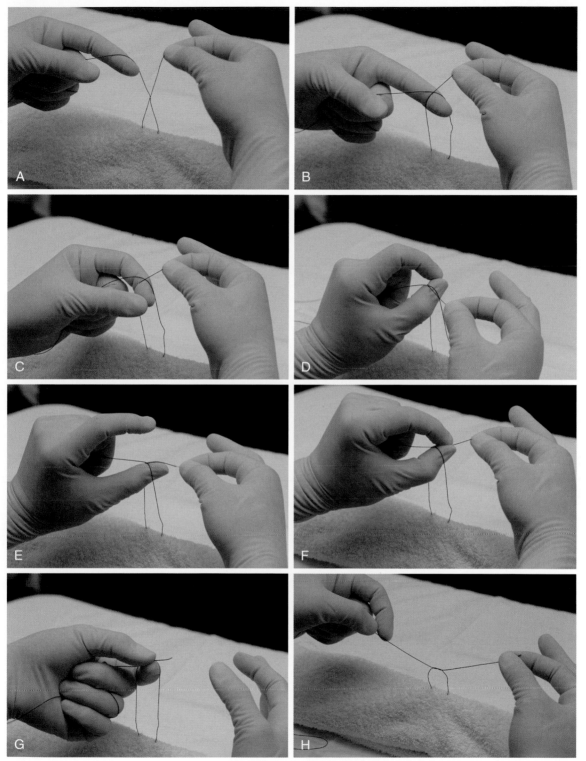

Fig. 7.32 Two-handed surgical knot

Continued

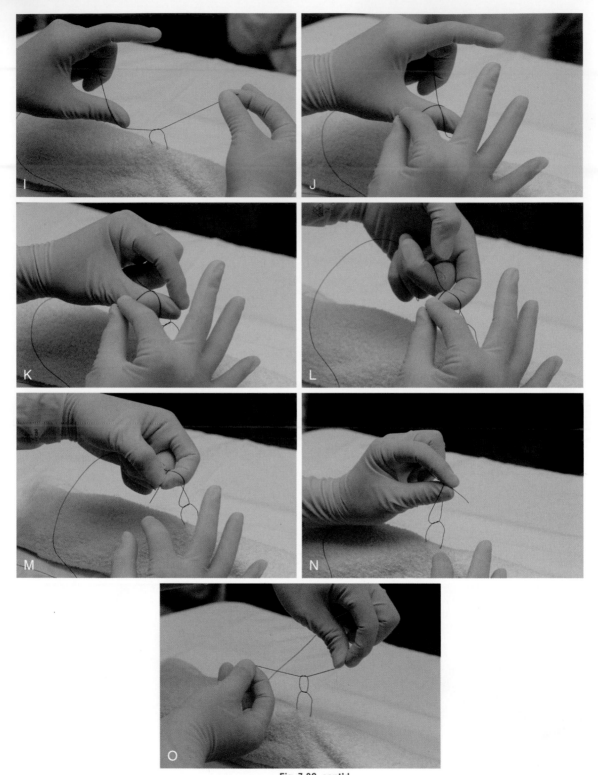

Fig. 7.32, cont'd

to complete a square knot. The suture is first grasped in the palm of the left hand. It is then placed over the index finger of that hand, which acts as a bridge for the suture material. The right hand grasps the other end of the suture material between the thumb and index finger in a pincer grip (Fig. 7.32A). The right hand is then used to bring the suture between the left thumb and index finger (Fig. 7.32B). After closing the left thumb and index fingers through the loop of suture material (Fig. 7.32C), the wrist is pronated, bringing the suture material that was originally over the index finger to now rest over the thumb (Fig. 7.32D). The right hand is then used to cross its suture material over the strand being supported by the left thumb (Fig. 7.32E), and this is then grasped between the index finger and thumb of the left hand (Fig. 7.32F). After releasing the suture with the right hand, the left hand is supinated, bringing the second strand of suture material under the first (Fig. 7.32G). Horizontal tension is applied to each strand of suture material, making the knot taut (Fig. 7.32H). This completes the first overhand half hitch of the square knot.

Grasping the same sides of the suture material with each hand as before, the suture is now brought over the thumb of the left hand, as opposed to the index finger as before (Fig. 7.32I). The right hand again brings its suture material between the thumb and index finger of the left hand (Fig. 7.32J). Closing the fingers around this loop of

suture (Fig. 7.32K), the left hand is supinated through the loop (Fig. 7.32L). The left thumb and index finger then grasp the suture from the right hand (Fig. 7.32M). The left hand is pronated, bringing the suture material through the loop (Fig. 7.32N). Again, horizontal tension is placed on each strand of the suture material, but this time in the opposite direction of the first (Fig. 7.32O). This brings the knot down, completing the second half hitch of the square knot. Additional alternating throws may be performed to add security to the knot.

One-Handed Knots

One-handed knots (Fig. 7.33) are an alternative to two-handed knots in certain situations. They may be useful when tension needs to be kept on one end of suture material to prevent the tissues from pulling apart. This technique is also helpful in cases where a narrow space prevents two hands from completing a tie. These knots are also typically faster to perform than two-handed surgical knots. However, one-handed ties may allow knot loosening if proper technique is not used. They do not allow for as great a tension to be generated on each throw as a two-handed tie does.

To perform a one-handed tie, the palm of the left hand grasps the suture material and then it is placed over the extended index finger of that hand. The right hand grasps the other end of the suture material between the thumb and index finger (Fig. 7.33A).

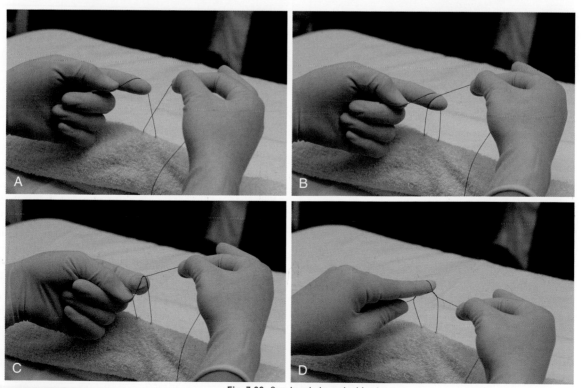

Fig. 7.33 One-handed surgical knot

Continued

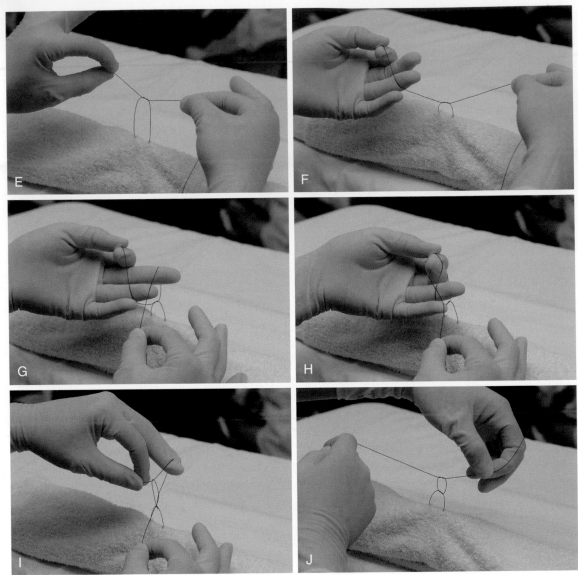

Fig. 7.33, cont'd

The right hand brings its suture across the suture being held over the left index finger, and the left index finger hooks the right hand's suture (Fig. 7.33B). Of note, the thumb of the left hand can be used to displace the suture being held by the left hand outward. The distal phalanx of the left index finger is then extended, passing under its original suture material (Fig. 7.33C). This allows it to be pulled through the loop of suture that was just created by extending the left index finger (Fig. 7.33D). Horizontal tension is then placed on each end of the suture to complete the first half hitch of the square knot (Fig. 7.33E).

Now holding the end of the suture material between the thumb and index finger of the left hand, the suture is brought across the palm of the hand and hooked around either the fourth or fifth digit of the left hand (Fig. 7.33F). The suture held in the right hand is brought over the suture held in the left hand, in a direction toward the surgeon (Fig. 7.33G). The middle finger of the left hand hooks this suture and brings it down below the suture held in the left hand (Fig. 7.33H). The middle finger of the left hand is then extended at the same time the left hand is pronated, bringing the suture held by the left hand beneath the other suture end (Fig. 7.33I). The suture material is then released by the thumb and index finger of the left hand as the middle finger draws it through the loop. Regrasping both ends of the suture, horizontal tension is placed on each end to complete the second half hitch of the square knot (Fig. 7.33J).

Instrument Tying

An instrument, typically a needle driver, may also be used to perform a square knot. This is frequently done,

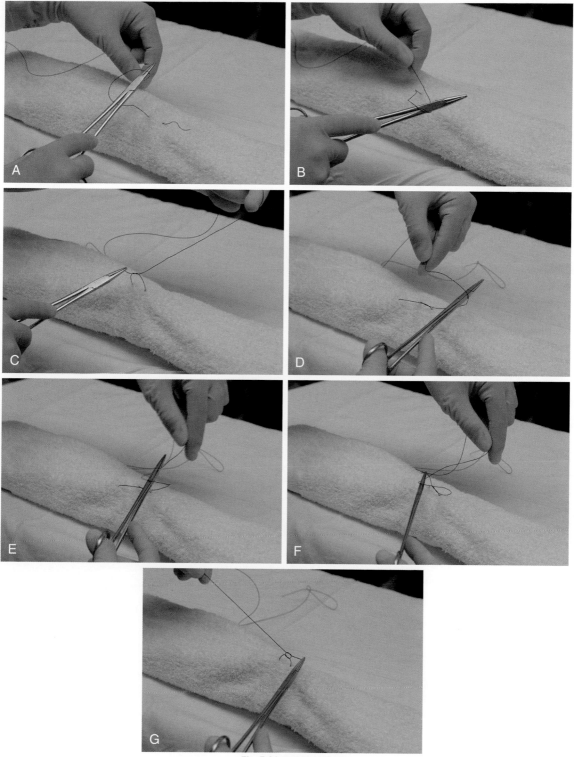

Fig. 7.34 Instrument tying

as it can quickly complete a surgical knot and requires less suture material to perform than a hand-thrown knot. The nondominant hand is used to grasp one end of the suture material. This is typically the longer end with the needle on it if the suture was just placed through tissue.

The suture is wrapped around the end of the instrument in a clockwise fashion (Fig. 7.34A). The tip of the instrument is used to grasp the other end of the suture material (Fig. 7.34B). It is then pulled back through the loop to complete the first half hitch of the square knot as horizontal tension is placed on each end of the suture (Fig. 7.34C). It should be noted that the suture should be in the correct orientation at this point to allow the knot to lie flat.

The suture material is then wrapped around the instrument in a counterclockwise fashion (Fig. 7.34D–E). Again, the instrument is used to grasp the other end of the suture and pull it back through the loop (Fig. 7.34F). Placing horizontal tension on each end of the suture material, the knot is laid down, completing the second half hitch of the square knot (Fig. 7.34G). Additional throws of the suture in alternating directions add security to the surgical knot.

CHAPTER 8
MAKING AN INCISION

Making an incision is a fundamental aspect of surgical practice, allowing access to pathology that can be addressed through structural manipulation. Whether it is draining an abscess, removing a tumor, or bypassing an obstructed vessel or visceral organ, the skin and underlying tissues must be traversed. Although many endoscopic procedures do not require cutting the skin, most surgical procedures will require at least one incision. Each surgical procedure requires a unique surgical plan. This chapter focuses on incision planning and how to make surgical incisions.

PLANNING THE INCISION—WHERE AND HOW LONG

The decision as to where and how long to make an incision depends on the intended surgical procedure, the extent to which the pathology is known, the method of the procedure, and the acuity of the surgery. Whereas an incision for a thyroidectomy will be relatively small and delicate, the incision for a lower extremity amputation will be much larger. Additionally, a laparoscopic appendectomy requires small incisions to be made at sites somewhat distant from the right lower quadrant of the abdomen, where the appendix is located, whereas an open appendectomy dictates that an incision be made in the right lower quadrant of the abdomen near the appendix. In contrast, when a suspected small bowel obstruction occurs in which the site of obstruction is uncertain, a vertical midline incision is commonly made to provide exposure to the entire intestine.

In general, incisions are made as small as possible to accomplish the intended procedure. This allows a more favorable cosmetic outcome following the surgery, facilitates faster wound healing, and decreases evaporative fluid losses. In many instances the use of handheld and self-retaining retractors can provide sufficient exposure to the operative site; however, minimizing incision size should not take precedence over ensuring optimal access to pathology. Therefore, in some cases an incision may need to be extended to provide optimal visualization of the target structures.

A unique consideration for incision size is that of laparoscopic and robotic surgeries. Using small incisions and ports placed through these incisions, a wide pallet of instruments can be utilized to perform a surgery. Although the size and type of pathology can differ greatly, port sizes are relatively constant and range in size by only a few millimeters. For example, a laparoscopic cholecystectomy requires the same size port incisions to be made as a laparoscopic colon resection. It is important to note, however, that the number of ports, location of ports, and size of the extraction site will vary based on the type of surgery being performed.

Most open surgical procedures will dictate that the skin incision be made over the organ or area of interest. However, this may be modified based on the location of previous surgical scars and with the intent of minimizing postoperative pain. Several studies have demonstrated that a transverse or oblique incision may decrease the incidence of postoperative incisional pain and increase respiratory effort, especially in the immediate postoperative period.[1-3] The ability to access the intended surgical site should not be compromised, however, in an effort to make an incision over a previous surgical scar or minimize pain.

A variety of standardized surgical incisions have been described based on the intended surgery and location of pathology. Although deviations from these incisions may occur based on patient body habitus, their uses have been found to offer optimal surgical site exposure, decrease morbidity, and provide for optimal cosmetic outcomes.

Surgeries of the Chest
Median Sternotomy

Incisions for surgeries of the chest are primarily composed of two different types: the median sternotomy and thoracotomy. The median sternotomy provides excellent exposure for cardiac surgery, as well as bilateral pulmonary, trachea, bronchi, and mediastinal surgeries. It has long been considered the gold standard for open cardiac surgery.[4] An incision is made from the sternal notch to a point a few centimeters below

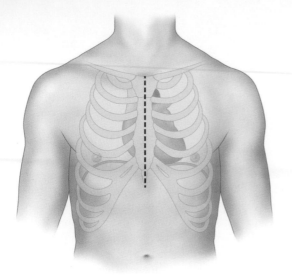

Fig. 8.1 Median sternotomy incision

the xiphoid process using a surgical knife (Fig. 8.1). Dissection is carried down to the mediastinum by dividing the sternum in the midline with an oscillating saw. The incision is kept open during surgery via use of a retractor. This incision has been shown to provide excellent exposure and allows for minimal postoperative complications such as wound infection and breakdown.

Thoracotomy Incision

A thoracotomy incision is the incision of choice for most open thoracic surgeries, including pulmonary lobectomy and pneumonectomy. An incision is typically made in the intercostal space and may be extended to allow enough exposure to the operative site (Fig. 8.2). Dissection is carried down into the pleural space, and a retractor is used to aid in providing exposure between the ribs. These incisions tend to result in a significant amount of postoperative pain and may serve as a cause of postoperative morbidity, given that patients tend to be restricted in their ability to breath effectively, resulting in atelectasis and pneumonia.

Surgeries of the Abdomen
Midline Incision

A wide variety of abdominal incision types exist, each aimed at providing optimal exposure of the operative site while minimizing morbidity associated with the incision. The midline incision is one of the most common and variable surgical incisions of the abdomen. Depending on the operative site, upper midline, lower midline, and extended midline incisions may be utilized (Fig. 8.3). Upper midline incisions typically

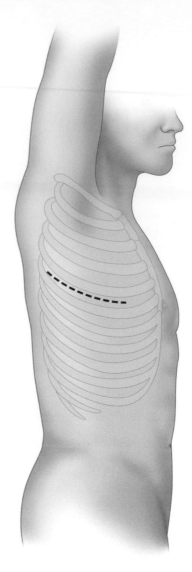

Fig. 8.2 Thoracotomy incision

extend from the inferior border of the xiphoid process to a point just above the umbilicus. Lower midline incisions extend from a point just below the umbilicus to the pubic symphysis. Each of these incisions can be carried inferiorly or superiorly, respectively, to allow adequate exposure. When an incision is to extend past the umbilicus, typically a smooth curve is made around this landmark and carried back along in the midline superiorly and inferiorly.

Chevron Incision

The Chevron incision is a large, upper abdominal incision that allows exposure to the liver, pancreas, and other upper abdominal structures. The incision is initiated in the midaxillary line under the ribs on one side of

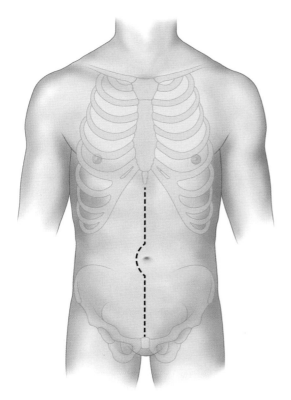

Fig. 8.3 Midline incisions

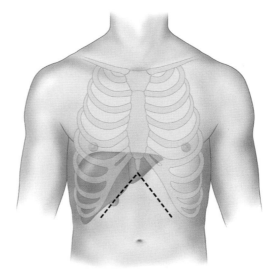

Fig. 8.4 Chevron incision

the abdomen and is carried under the ribs and xiphoid process to the contralateral midaxillary line (Fig. 8.4). The midline point of the incision can also be used as the lower point of a median sternotomy incision during surgeries that require a combined abdominal and thoracic approach.

Thoracoabdominal Incision

The thoracoabdominal incision provides excellent exposure to the thoracic, abdominal, and retroperitoneal compartments (Fig. 8.5). It is particularly useful in cases that necessitate exposure of the esophagus, gastroesophageal junction, stomach, pancreas, kidney, adrenal gland, or great vessels. As a large incision is necessary, and two separate body cavities are opened, the incidence of postoperative complications may be increased.[5]

Flank Incision

The flank incision offers access to the retroperitoneum without entering the intraperitoneal cavity (Fig. 8.6). The patient is typically placed in the lateral flank position, and the table is flexed with the kidney rest elevated to open the space between the ribs and the iliac crest. An incision is made to extend from the superior margin of the 10th, 11th, or 12th rib to the anterior midline. This incision provides excellent exposure for

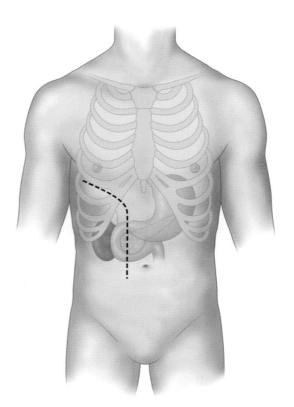

Fig. 8.5 Thoracoabdominal incision

adrenal, renal, ureteral, and other retroperitoneal surgeries. Sometimes a portion of a rib may need to be resected. Flank incisions have been associated with some patients experiencing a flank bulge postoperatively, likely due to intercostal nerve injury at the time of the procedure.[6]

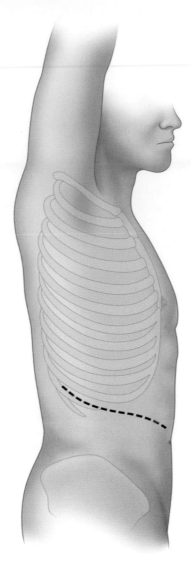

Fig. 8.6 Flank incision

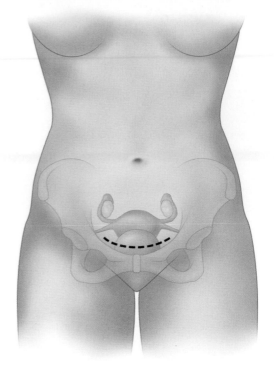

Fig. 8.7 Pfannenstiel incision

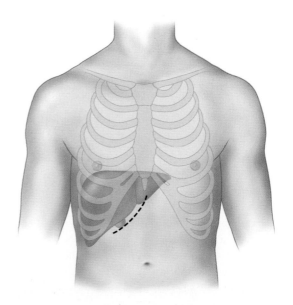

Fig. 8.8 Kocher incision

Pfannenstiel Incision

The Pfannenstiel incision is a transverse incision made in the lower abdomen approximately 1–2 cm superior to the pubic symphysis (Fig. 8.7). After incising the skin for approximately 10 to 15 cm, the subcutaneous tissues are entered transversely. Typically, the anterior rectus sheath is then entered transversely and the underlying rectus muscle is bluntly dissected off, thereafter separating the muscle at the midline raphe. The transversalis fascia and posterior rectus sheath are then entered vertically to gain access to the abdominal cavity. The Pfannenstiel incision has long been the incision of choice for cesarean section and is often used in other pelvic surgeries, such as hysterectomy and bladder surgeries. It provides excellent cosmetic outcomes and can often be concealed below the bikini line.

Kocher Incision

A Kocher incision is an incision made in the right upper quadrant of the abdomen, typically used for open cholecystectomy (Fig. 8.8). It is a curvilinear incision that provides exposure to the gallbladder and biliary tract, and limited exposure to the liver. With the rise of laparoscopic cholecystectomy and

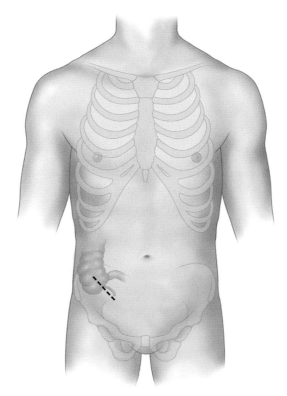

Fig. 8.9 McBurney incision

decreased morbidity as compared to open cholecystectomy, the use of this incision has dramatically decreased.

McBurney Incision

The McBurney incision is an oblique incision made at McBurney's point (approximately one-third of the distance from the anterior superior iliac spine to the umbilicus (Fig. 8.9). First described in 1894 by Charles McBurney, it provides excellent exposure for an appendectomy and was the standard of care prior to the advent of the laparoscopic appendectomy.[7] Today, as with the Kocher incision, the McBurney incision is seldom used.

LOCAL ANESTHESIA

Local anesthesia is often given during surgical procedures. It may be administered alone to temporarily reduce pain during and after a procedure, such as is done during minor procedures like an incision and drainage of a skin abscess, or in combination with general anesthesia. It is best given *prior* to an incision being initiated to reduce pain.

Local anesthetics are primarily composed of two groups: amides and esters. Amides, which are more commonly used, include lidocaine (Xylocaine), mepivacaine (Carbocaine, Isocaine), bupivacaine (Marcaine,

Sensorcaine), etidocaine (Duranest), and ropivacaine (Naropin). Esters, which are less commonly used secondary to a historically greater incidence of allergic reactions and greater toxicity, include procaine (Novocaine), tetracaine, cocaine, and benzocaine.[8-10]

Anesthetic agents can be combined with epinephrine to provide local vasoconstriction. This allows for less periprocedural bleeding, reduces absorption of the anesthetic agent into the circulation, and prolongs the duration of action of the anesthetic agent. The use of epinephrine with a local anesthetic agent may be contraindicated, however, in patients with severe peripheral arterial disease, when being used on sites with end arteries such as digits or the penis, or when the amount of anesthetic agent is great and the patient has an underlying condition that may be exacerbated by epinephrine (e.g., severe hypertension, pheochromocytoma, or hyperthyroidism), although this dogma may be changing.[11,12]

Table 8.1 provides a comparison of four of the most commonly used local anesthetics. The choice of an anesthetic depends on patient-related factors, such as whether the patient has experienced a previous allergic reaction after administration of an anesthetic agent, as well as procedure-related factors, including the length of the procedure and the need for rapid onset of action. When being used during short procedures, administration of the local anesthetic at the beginning of the procedure usually is sufficient to provide a great enough duration of anesthesia. When being used for procedures that require a greater amount of time, it may be advisable to administer an additional dose of a local anesthetic at the conclusion of the procedure.

Anesthetic agents typically come in defined concentrations in glass or plastic vials of premixed solution. The amount of local anesthetic agent necessary for a procedure should be determined, and that amount should be drawn into a syringe. Using a 10-cc or smaller syringe allows the anesthetic agent to easily be injected into the subcutaneous layer of the skin and is therefore recommended. To draw the anesthetic agent into the syringe, a large needle, typically 18 gauge (G), is connected to the syringe, and air is drawn into the syringe (Fig. 8.10A). The needle is inserted through the diaphragm of the vial, then air is injected into the vial (Fig. 8.10B). This increases the pressure in the vial so that the anesthetic agent will easily flow back into the syringe (Fig. 8.10C). The needle should then be withdrawn from the vial and exchanged for a smaller needle (typically 25, 27, or 30 G) that will be used for injection (Fig. 8.10D). When doing this in a sterile manner, a nonsterile individual presents the vial of anesthetic to a sterile individual holding the syringe. The sterile needle is inserted through the diaphragm of the vial. All other parts of the vial other

Table 8.1 Comparison of Commonly Used Anesthetic Agents for Local Anesthesia

| Infiltration Anesthetic | Concentration (%) | Physiochemical Properties | | | | Maximum Allowable Dose[a] | | Maximum Total Dose[a] |
		Lipid:Water Solubility	Relative Potency	Onset of Action (min)	Duration (min)	mg/kg	mL/kg	mg Equivalent Solution Volume
Lidocaine								
Without epinephrine	1	2.9	2	2–5	50–120	4–5	0.4–0.5	300 30 mL of 1%
With epinephrine (1:200,000)	1	2.9	2	2–5	60–180	5–7	0.5–0.7	500 50 mL of 1%
Mepivacaine								
Without epinephrine	1	0.8	2	2–5	50–120	5	0.5	300 30 mL of 1%
With epi-nephrine[b] (1:200,000)	1	0.8	2	2–5	60–180	5–7	0.5–0.7	500 50 mL of 1%
Bupivacaine								
Without epinephrine	0.25	27.5	8	5–10	240–480	2	0.8	175 70 mL of 0.25%
With epinephrine (1:200,000)	0.25	27.5	8	5–10	240–480	3	1.2	225 90 mL of 0.25%
Procaine[c]	1	0.6	1	5–10	60–90	7–10	0.7–1.0	500 50 mL of 1%

[a]The maximum total dose for intradermal-subcutaneous infiltration anesthesia may vary according to the site of administration and concomitant use of vasoconstrictors. The maximum dosing values in this table are at the lower end of what many experts regard as safe. Lower doses and concentrations than what are listed are generally used for children, debilitated patients, or those with cardiac disease. Note that preparations of infiltrated local anesthetics are available in concentrations other than those shown in table. Maximum allowable and maximum total volumes shown apply only to the specific concentration of the preparation in the table. Toxicity may occur with doses within the suggested range, especially with inadvertent vascular injection.
[b]Not commercially available; provider must mix.
[c]Not commercially available in the United States or Canada.
Modified from Hsu D. Subcutaneous infiltration of local anesthetics. In: Stack A, Walls R, Miller S, eds. UpToDate. https://www.uptodate.com/contents/subcutaneous-infiltration-of-local-anesthetics

than the diaphragm should be considered nonsterile and should not be touched by the sterile individual. In the operative field, the circulating nurse often pours the agent in a sterile manner into a cup. The scrub technician then labels the cup with a pen to identify contents.

To administer a local anesthetic agent, the needle should be inserted just beneath the skin. In areas in which large blood vessels are present, drawing back on the syringe and ensuring no blood return prevents inadvertent injection of anesthetic into the systemic circulation. If a flash of blood is encountered when drawing back, the needle should be drawn back and redirected. Once the needle has been advanced underneath the skin, the anesthetic agent should be injected to produce a skin wheal while drawing back on the needle (Fig. 8.11). For incisions of sufficient length that require multiple needle sticks to produce adequate anesthesia, introducing the needle through a site that has already received the local anesthetic may reduce pain from the needle stick. Video 8.1. demonstrates how to correctly draw up a local anesthetic agent for injection and how to administer it.

HOW TO MAKE INCISIONS

A surgical incision consists of the cuts that are needed to access an area of interest to accomplish a surgical procedure. This may be as minor as incising skin to remove a skin lesion or as complex as incising skin, subcutaneous tissue, muscle, fascia, and the peritoneum to access the abdominal cavity. Skin incisions can be made with a knife blade or electrocautery. Fig. 8.12 shows the various blades available. In general, a #10 blade (Fig. 8.12A) is the standard blade used for long incisions, as well as to incise thicker, scarred tissue. A #15 blade is a smaller, more precise version of the #10 blade that is used to make smaller incisions (Fig. 8.12B). The #20 blade is a larger version of the #10 blade and is often used in orthopedic surgery cases (Fig. 8.12C). The #11 blade is useful for making a stab incision via its long narrow pointed tip (Fig. 8.12D). Sometimes a specialized hook blade may be needed to catch a structure and pull upward to transect tissue.

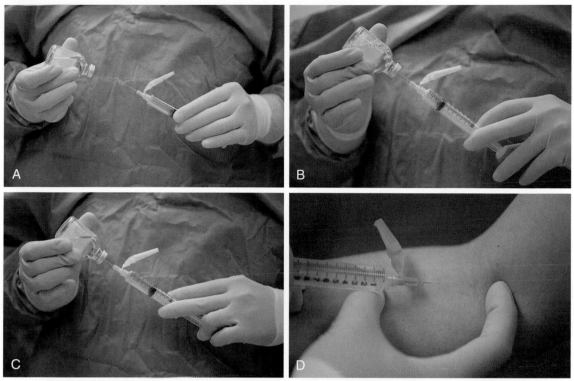

Fig. 8.10 Preparation of an anesthetic agent for injection. A. Air is drawn into a syringe with a preloaded large-gauge needle. B. The needle is inserted through the diaphragm of the vial, then air is injected. C. The anesthetic agent is then drawn into the syringe. D. A small-gauge needle is used for injection of the anesthetic agent into the skin.

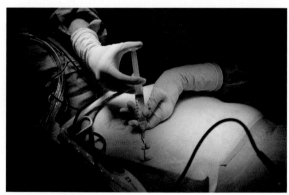

Fig. 8.11 Injecting local anesthetic agent

Skin

Skin incisions are typically performed with a skin knife. Different scalpel blades can be used based on incision length and tissue characteristics, such as skin thickness and the presence of scar tissue. The knife should to be held as in Video 8.2 and is placed perpendicular to the skin. This prevents skiving and beveling skin edges to help with an easier skin reapproximation and results in improved cosmetic outcomes.

To initiate a skin incision, the belly of the blade is rested on the skin surface (Fig. 8.13). Gentle pressure may be applied to the knife handle to allow it to cut through the epidermis. A controlled incision is made, preferably without lifting the blade to prevent jagged skin edges that are more difficult to close. Some surgeons continue the cut with the skin blade through the subcutaneous fat, although many use electrocautery, as it allows for controlled hemostasis.

It was initially believed that the use of the CUT function of electrocautery to make a skin incision resulted in worse postoperative wound healing, increased postoperative pain, and decreased cosmetic outcomes as compared to incision with a scalpel. The results of a several studies, however, dispel these notions, finding that wound healing is similar, there is no increase in the risk of infection, cosmetic outcomes do not differ, and patient satisfaction is unaffected. Additionally, incision time is decreased when using electrocautery, and blood loss is reduced.[13-16] Therefore, it is safe and effective to use electrocautery to make a skin incision.

Muscle

Incisions in muscle are typically performed with electrocautery. Whenever possible, it is advisable to bluntly split muscle along the direction of the fibers rather than incising tissue, as this results in less pain

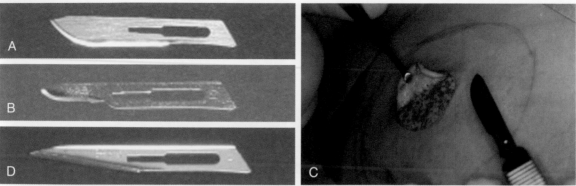

Fig. 8.12 Comparison between different scalpel blades. A. #10 blade. B. #15 blade. C. #20 blade. D. #11 blade. A,B,D, From Bhatia AC and Taneja A. Surgical instruments. In: Vidimos A, et al., eds., *Dermatologic Surgery.* Philadelphia: Elsevier, 2009. Print. C, From Hintschich, C, Altan-Yaycioglu, R. Management of post-enucleation socket syndrome. In: Spaeth GL, et al., eds., *Ophthalmic Surgery: Principles and Practice.* Philadelphia: Elsevier, 2012: 450-461. © 2012.

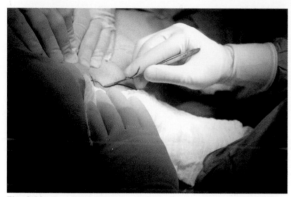

Fig. 8.13 Use of the belly of a #10 blade to perform a skin incision

and improved strength of the muscle. This is typically done during longitudinal abdominal incisions in the midline at the linea alba. When incising a muscle is necessary, care should be taken to try to reapproximate the two ends of the cut muscle fascicle during closure.

Muscle has an extremely rich vascular supply, and often even when using COAG electrocautery, bleeding is inevitable. Gently touching the bleeding muscle with the electrocautery pen, or grasping it with a forceps and touching the electrocautery pen to the forceps, is sufficient to stop the bleeding. However, sometimes a simple suture may be necessary to control persistent bleeding.

Fascia

In most surgical cases, the fascia is incised using electrocautery. Since fascia serves as the eventual strength layer during closure, it is important to attempt to make a clean cut for the purpose of simplifying closure, as well as maintaining the strength

of this layer. Cleaning the fascial layer of overlying tissue, either by sweeping it away with a surgical sponge or clearing it with a handheld retractor, may allow for easier fascial closure at the end of the procedure.

It is important when incising fascia to avoid past pointing with the tip of the electrocautery device. By inadvertently doing so, underlying structures such as bowel are at risk of thermal injury. For this reason, after making a small nick in the fascia, an instrument such as a Kelly clamp may be inserted and used to elevate the fascia off underlying structures so that it can be safely incised. In surgical cases in which a large amount of adhesions is expected, such as in patients who have had previous abdominal surgeries, a scissors may be used to incise the fascia until it is certain that there are no underlying adhesive bands of bowel or other organs that would be at risk of injury.

HEMOSTASIS

Achieving hemostasis is important during all steps of a surgical procedure. During an initial surgical incision, it is important to achieve hemostasis for several reasons. First, even small bleeding vessels can result in large blood loss if not recognized and addressed until the end of a major procedure. Second, bleeding from a surgical incision typically runs into the surgical field and can obscure vision of the field and be mistaken for bleeding from the surgical site. Third, even minor bleeding can result in large areas of skin bruising, thus distressing patients. Fourth, bleeding can lead to hematomas, which may become infected and compromise the surgical incision and closure.

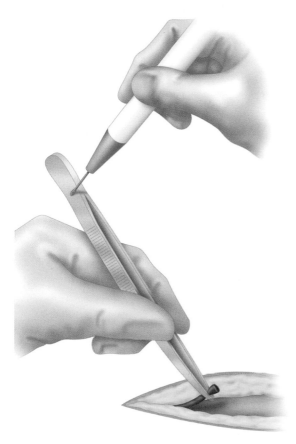

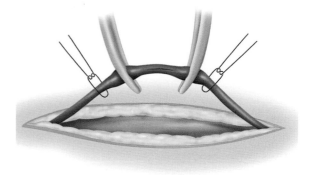

Fig. 8.15 Ligating a bleeding vessel with a surgical tie requires placing a tie beneath the clamped vessel.

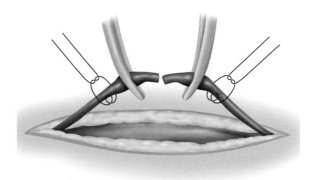

Fig. 8.16 Suture ligating a bleeding vessel requires throwing a suture beneath the vessel and performing a surgical tie.

Fig. 8.14 Grasping a bleeding vessel with a forceps and applying electrocautery to the forceps often causes the bleeding to stop.

Cautery

Most bleeding that occurs during the initial incision of a surgical procedure can be addressed with the COAG function of electrocautery. Simply touching the area of bleeding, or with more persistent bleeding, painting the area of concern, usually causes the bleeding to stop. For discrete areas of bleeding with larger vessels or more brisk bleeding that is thought to be arterial in nature, grasping the vessel with a forceps and touching the cautery pen to the forceps usually results in adequate hemostasis (Fig. 8.14).

Tie

In cases of bleeding in which the vessel is larger than can be controlled with electrocautery, placing a tie around the vessel may be necessary. To do this, the end of the vessel is grasped with a ratcheted instrument, such as a curved or right-angle clamp. If bleeding does not cease or significantly diminish after grasping the vessel, an attempt to gain better control of the vessel is necessary. After gaining adequate control of the bleeding vessel

with the clamp, a surgical tie is placed underneath the clamp and secured to control the vessel (Fig. 8.15). Different sizes of ties may be used depending on the size of the vessel, although the material used is typically an absorbable, braided suture.

Suture Ligation

In the case of persistent bleeding where a feeding blood vessel is apparent, suture ligating the vessel may be necessary. To do this, a suture is passed through the vessel at a site proximal to the bleeding, and an additional throw of the suture is placed around the vessel. (Fig. 8.16). If the vessel being ligated is the source of bleeding, this should stop when a surgical tie is thrown. In some cases, a figure-of-eight tie needs to be thrown to achieve hemostasis. This method of hemostasis is similar to placing a surgical tie with free suture material, differing only in that a suture must be thrown through the vessel to be ligated. As with placing a free tie, an absorbable, braided suture material is typically chosen.

REFERENCES

1. Bickenbach KA, Karanicolas PJ, Ammori JB, et al. Up and down or side to side? A systematic review and meta-analysis examining the impact of incision on outcomes after abdominal surgery. *American Journal of Surgery.* 2013;206(3):400–409.
2. Brown SR, Goodfellow PB. Transverse verses midline incisions for abdominal surgery. *Cochrane Database of Systematic Reviews.* 2005;(4):CD005199.
3. Inaba T, Okinaga K, Fukushima R, et al. Prospective randomized study of two laparotomy incisions for gastrectomy: midline incision versus transverse incision. *Gastric Cancer.* 2004;7(3):167–171.
4. Reser D, Caliskan E, Tolboom H, Guidotti A, Maisano F. Median sternotomy. *Multimedia Manual of Cardiothoracic Surgery.* 2015. pii:mmv017.
5. Lumsden AB, Colborn GL, Sreeram S, Skandalakis LJ. The surgical anatomy and technique of the thoracoabdominal incision. *Surgical Clinics of North America.* 1993;73(4):633–644.
6. Chatterjee S, Nam R, Fleshner N, Klotz L. Permanent flank bulge is a consequence of flank incision for radical nephrectomy in one half of patients. *Urologic Oncology.* 2004;22(1):36–39.
7. McBurney CIV. The incision made in the abdominal wall in cases of appendicitis, with a description of a new method of operating. *Annals of Surgery.* 1894;20(1):38–43.
8. Achar S, Kundu S. Principles of office anesthesia: part I. Infiltrative anesthesia. *American Family Physician.* 2002;66(1):91–94.
9. Ahlstrom KK, Frodel JL. Local anesthetics for facial plastic procedures. *Otolaryngologic Clinics of North America.* 2002;35(1):29–53. v-vi.
10. Tetzlaff JE. The pharmacology of local anesthetics. *Anesthesiology Clinics of North America.* 2000;18(2):217–233. v.
11. Krunic AL, Wang LC, Soltani K, Weitzul S, Taylor RS. Digital anesthesia with epinephrine: an old myth revisited. *Journal of the American Academy of Dermatology.* 2004;51(5):755–759.
12. Prabhakar H, Rath S, Kalaivani M, Bhanderi N. Adrenaline with lidocaine for digital nerve blocks. *Cochrane Database of Systematic Reviews.* 2015;(3):CD010645.
13. Aird LN, Brown CJ. Systematic review and meta-analysis of electrocautery versus scalpel for surgical skin incisions. *American Journal of Surgery.* 2012;204(2):216–221.
14. Chau JK, Dzigielewski P, Mlynarek A, et al. Steel scalpel versus electrocautery blade: comparison of cosmetic and patient satisfaction outcomes of different incision methods. *Journal of Otolaryngology—Head and Neck Surgery.* 2009;38(4):427–433.
15. Kearns SR, Connolly EM, McNally S, McNamara DA, Deasy J. Randomized clinical trial of diathermy versus scalpel incision in elective midline laparotomy. *British Journal of Surgery.* 2001;88(1):41–44.
16. Stupart DA, Sim FW, Chan ZH, Guest GD, Watters DA. Cautery versus scalpel for abdominal skin incisions: a double blind, randomized crossover trial of scar cosmesis. *ANZ Journal of Surgery.* 2016;86(4):303–306.

CHAPTER 9

PUTTING EVERYTHING BACK TOGETHER: CONCLUDING THE OPERATION

Once surgical pathology has been addressed through the performance of an operation, efforts need to be made to ensure that manipulated tissue is restored as closely as possible to conditions prior to the surgery. Care needs to be taken to do a final inspection of the operative site and then reconstruct tissue in a step-by-step manner. It is also important to note that dressings need to be applied that are effective in protecting both the wound and the environment, including healthcare workers and other individuals.

INSPECTING THE FIELD

Adequate hemostasis is critical to surgical recovery. Even small amounts of bleeding into a large potential space can be problematic. Unrecognized bleeding can result in postoperative hemodynamic instability and concomitant effects on other organs. Moreover, a postoperative hematoma provides for a site of potential infection. Additionally, the hematoma can be distressing for patients if it causes a visible bulge or ecchymosis. If blood is pooling at the surgical site, one must evaluate the wound to determine if it is from the operative site or runs down from the incision or adjacent tissue.

To inspect for hemostasis, the first step is to visually examine the immediate operative site. Arterial bleeding will manifest as brisk, bright red blood welling into the operative field; however, slow venous oozing may not be quite as apparent. It may be difficult to discern whether a small amount of blood in the field is simply leftover from the procedure or truly represents a significant active bleed. Additionally, when slow oozing is manifest, at times it is more harmful to try to stop it than allowing it to cease on its own. This is certainly the case when bleeding is suspected near vital organs, nerves, and major blood vessels, in which cautery and hemostatic agents could potentially be harmful.

One should also inspect for any inadvertent, unnoticed collateral injuries caused during the procedure. During the course of a procedure in which the focus is in the immediate working operative space, injuries can occur that may go unrecognized until later. Retractors or errant discharge of electrocautery could cause unsuspected injuries. Injury may also occur while introducing instruments into the operative field. This is especially relevant during laparoscopic and robotic surgeries, in which instruments are introduced without visual guidance. Although rare, ischemia from anesthesia and hypoperfusion can occur, and therefore the viability of tissue should be assessed. All viscera, organs, and surrounding tissue should undergo a thorough visual inspection, as unrecognized injuries can lead to repeat surgical exploration, significant morbidity, and even death.

IRRIGATION

After performing a visual dry inspection of the operative field, the wound should be irrigated with a sterile solution. This is usually performed with either normal saline or sterile water, although in cases that involve contaminated wounds, such as orthopedic injuries and penetrating trauma, a chlorhexidine-containing solution may be used. Antibiotic-containing solutions are typically not used, as they provide little added benefit, except in cases in which implants have been placed.[1,2]

The purpose of wound irrigation is twofold. First, it allows for further assessment of bleeding. Bleeding that may not have been appreciated in a dry field may be seen through the clear irrigant solution as a red stream. This is aided by using sterile water as the irrigant, as red blood cells lyse in water, thereby allowing them to be seen more easily. Second, wound irrigation serves to remove blood clots, foreign bodies, microbes, and debris from the operative site.[3] Clearing the wound promotes healing and reduces the incidence of surgical site infection (SSI).[1,4]

To irrigate a wound, the irrigating solution is usually poured into the field and then suctioned out. This may be performed more than once in contaminated or dirty wounds. During laparoscopic and robotic surgeries, a suction irrigator device may be used to sequentially irrigate the wound and then suction out the irrigation fluid. In particularly dirty wounds, such as those of orthopedic injuries and penetrating trauma, a pulsed lavage irrigator may be used to more effectively cleanse the wound. For large open wounds, the irrigation fluid should be warmed to minimize the risk of lowering core body temperature.

HEMOSTASIS AND HEMOSTATIC AGENTS

One of the foremost principles of surgical technique is ensuring adequate hemostasis at the conclusion of a procedure. This is achieved by using surgical clips, ties, and electrocautery, and, in some instances, adjunctive hemostatic agents. Hemostatic agents are synthetic topical materials that enhance local clotting of blood. Their use in patients who are receiving anticoagulation, have platelet dysfunction, or have a known bleeding diathesis may be helpful in controlling the slow ooze from raw tissue surfaces. They are not a substitute for good surgical technique but instead offer an adjunct to inadequate or impractical hemostasis. Hemostatic agents vary in both mechanism of action and cost. Table 9.1 presents a review of the different commercially available hemostatic agents.[5]

Hemostatic agents are available in both dry and biologically active liquid form, each being placed over the area requiring hemostasis. Each has specific uses, as well as advantages and disadvantages. Dry matrix agents in general are less expensive, typically in the range of $50 to $100 per application, as opposed to $300 to $750 per application for many of the biologically active agents. All agents come prepackaged for a single patient use. Depending on the situation, one package may be split to use over multiple areas of the operative field, or several packages and combinations of agents may be needed.

Dry Matrix Agents

Oxidized regenerated cellulose (SURGICEL, NU-KNIT, FIBRILLAR) is a plant-based hemostatic agent that is usually supplied as a mesh sheet (Fig. 9.1). It is pliable and easily manipulated into different forms, allowing it to be used in both open and laparoscopic surgeries. It is placed directly onto the site of oozing and acts by activating the coagulation cascade to promote blood clotting. It serves as a scaffold on which a thrombus can form and typically dissolves in 7 to 14 days.[6,7]

Absorbable gelatin matrix (GELFOAM, SURGI-FOAM) products are derived from porcine-based collagen and are supplied as a dry sponge material. When moistened, they are easily compressed and can be placed

Table 9.1 Commercially Available Hemostatic Agents

Category	Type	Commercial Name
Passive (i.e., mechanical)	Porcine gelatin	GELFOAM SURGIFOAM powder and sponge
	Bovine collagen	Avitene Helistat INSTAT Ultrafoam
	Oxidized regenerated cellulose	SURGICEL SURGICEL FIBRILLAR SURGICEL NU-KNIT
	Polysaccharide spheres	SURGICEL SNoW
	Beeswax, paraffin, isopropyl palmate	Arista Vitasure Bone wax
Active	Bovine thrombin	Thrombin-JMI
	Pooled human thrombin	EVITHROM
	Recombinant thrombin	Recothrom
Flowable	Bovine gelatin and pooled human thrombin	FLOSEAL
	Bovine gelatin (and/or thrombin)	SURGIFLO
Fibrin sealant	Pooled human plasma	EVICEL TISSEEL
	Patient's own plasma and bovine thrombin	Vitagel
	Patient's own plasma	Cryoseal
Adhesives	Polyethylene glycol hydrogels (PEG)	COSEAL
	PEG + trilysine amine	DuraSeal
	PEG + human serum albumin	Progel
	Liquid monomers	DERMABOND LiquiBand SurgiSeal
	Synthetic tissue sealants	OMNEX
	Glutaraldehyde cross linked with bovine albumin	BioGlue

GELFOAM and FLOSEAL are registered trademarks, and TISSEEL and COSEAL are trademarks of Baxter Corporation, Deerfield, IL. SURGIFOAM, INSTAT, SURGICEL, SURGICEL NU-KNIT, EVITHROM, SURGIFLO, EVICEL, and DERMABOND are registered trademarks, and SURGICEL FIBRILLAR, SURGICEL SNoW, and OMNEX are trademarks of Ethicon, Johnson & Johnson, Inc., Somerville, NJ. Avitene and Ultrafoam are trademarks of Davol, a Bard Company, Warwick, RI. Helistat is a registered trademark of Integra Life Sciences Corporation, Plainsboro, NJ. Arista is a trademark of Medafor, Minneapolis, MN. Vitasure is a registered trademark of Orthovita, Malvern, PA. Thrombin-JMI is a registered trademark of Pfizer, New York, NY. Recothrom is a registered trademark of The Medicines Company, Parsippany, NJ. Vitagel is a trademark of Stryker, Malvern, PA. Cryoseal is a registered trademark of ThermoGenesis Corporation, Rancho Cordova, CA. DuraSeal is a trademark of Covidien, Boulder, CO. Progel is a registered trademark of Neomend, Irvine, CA. LiquiBand is a registered trademark of Cardinal Health, Dublin, OH. SurgiSeal is a registered trademark of Adhezion Biomedical, Wyomissing, PA. BioGlue is a registered trademark of CryoLife, Kennesaw, GA. Used with permission from Camp MA. Hemostatic agents: a guide to safe practice for perioperative nurses. AORN Journal. 2014;100(2):131–147.

through laparoscopic ports and in other tight spaces. Similar to oxidized regenerated cellulose products, they promote the clotting cascade and allow a thrombus to form on the gelatin. These products typically dissolve

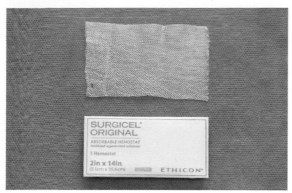

Fig. 9.1 Surgical hemostatic agent. © Ethicon 2017. Reproduced with permission.

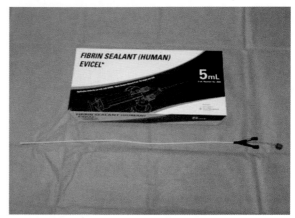

Fig. 9.3 TISSEEL hemostatic agent. From Masel JL, Transurethral use of Evicel® Fibrin Sealant. *Urol Case Rep.* 2016;4:5–7.

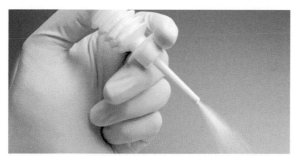

Fig. 9.2 Arista hemostatic agent. © 2012 C.R. Bard, Inc. Used with permission. Bard is a registered trademark of C.R. Bard, Inc.

in 4 to 6 weeks. They have been linked to an increased incidence of infection, potentially due to their long time to dissolution.[6–8]

Microporous polysaccharide spheres (Arista) are available in a powder-like form and are derived from plant-based starch material (Fig. 9.2). They act to absorb fluids, including blood plasma, which serves to concentrate platelets and proteins of the coagulation cascade. Application is by a bellows-type applicator in which the powder is applied to the surface. Microporous polysaccharide spheres can be used in conjunction with other hemostatic agents and are advantageous since they dissolve rapidly (within 24 to 48 hours) and present a very low risk of infection.[7,9]

Microfibrillar collagen (Avitene) is supplied in either a sheet or powder form and is derived from bovine collagen. Like other dry matrix agents, it serves as a scaffold on which proteins of the clotting cascade and platelets can form, activating the clotting cascade. It is placed directly onto the site of bleeding and typically is absorbed within 8 to 12 weeks.[7]

Biologically Active Agents

Topical thrombin agents (Thrombin-JMI, EVITHROM, Recothrom) are bovine- or human-derived liquid preparations that can be directly applied to areas of bleeding.

They are typically delivered via a syringe and needle-type applicator that allows them to be directed to the site at which they are needed. Topical thrombin agents may also be applied in conjunction with a gelatin matrix that allows for an immediate scaffold on which clot formation can occur. FLOSEAL and SURGIFLO are two commercially available preparations of thrombin/gelatin combinations that are frequently used. Topical thrombin agents also have the advantage of not being inhibited by urine. Additionally, they resist formation of urinary stones, whereas some dry matrix agents may act as a nidus for stone formation. These advantages allow topical thrombin agents to be used effectively in surgeries that involve entry into the urinary tract and make them a favored hemostatic agent during urologic surgeries.[7,10,11]

Fibrin sealants (TISSEEL, EVICEL, EVARREST) are human-derived solutions of fibrinogen, Factor XII, thrombin, and calcium that come as a liquid preparation (Fig. 9.3). They are stored frozen and come packaged as a two-component system, in which a solution of fibrinogen and Factor XII is stored in one syringe and thrombin and calcium in another. After being allowed to thaw, an applicator allows the two syringes to mix together as they are applied to the site of use. When combined, a fibrin-based clot forms that aids in hemostasis. Fibrin sealants have the advantage of being absorbed immediately and pose a low risk of infection.[6,7,12]

Bovine albumin-glutaraldehyde tissue adhesives (Bio-Glue) are albumin-based liquid preparations that are effective for moderate bleeding. They have received approval for use as a sealant for large vessels in cardiac surgery and may be effective at times when other hemostatic agents fail. When placed over a site of bleeding, these preparations form an adhesive matrix that results in hemostasis (Fig. 9.4).[7,13,14]

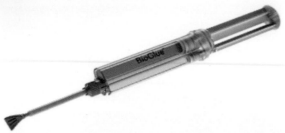

Fig. 9.4 BioGlue hemostatic agent. Used with permission from CryoLife, Inc.

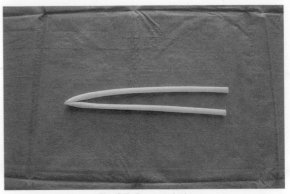

Fig. 9.5 Penrose drain

DRAINS

When to Drain

Surgical drains are placed after procedures for a variety of reasons. The most common is to prevent accumulation of fluid that could result in a nidus for infection. They are also used to reduce dead space, prevent increases in pressure that could disrupt surgical anastomoses or have untoward effects by compressing organs (e.g., the brain), and decrease pain from the collection of fluid. They are also placed in the setting of infection to prevent recurrence. Drains may also be placed if there is a suspected body fluid leak (i.e., urine, pancreatic fluid) to prevent reabsorption of electrolytes or local irritation. Drains may be either active, such as those that pull fluid through negative pressure suction, or passive, which allow fluid to drain by gravity.

Although usually safe and effective, complications from surgical drains do occur. They have the potential to introduce infection into a surgical wound and should therefore be removed when deemed no longer needed. In rare cases, they may allow for hernia formation or bleeding after removal. There have been instances when drains break upon removal due to tissue ingrowth or inadvertent suture fixation of the drain within the body. In these cases, surgical exploration may be needed for removal. Pain at the site of a drain, especially on removal, is a common patient complaint.

Types of Drains

Multiple different types of surgical drains are available, with each designed for a specific purpose. The following is a review of some of the most commonly used surgical drains.

Penrose

A Penrose drain is a soft, flexible rubber drain that passively allows fluid to drain from the surgical site (Fig. 9.5). It does not have a collection device and therefore empties into a surgical dressing. It is often placed in spaces such as subcutaneous fat to prevent fluid accumulation. This drain is often sutured in place with an air knot, and a safety pin is sometimes placed on the drain to prevent it from migrating into an incision. Penrose drains are an open system and potentially may introduce infection into a surgical wound.

Jackson-Pratt

A Jackson-Pratt (JP) drainage system consists of a grenade-shaped external bulb that is used to create negative pressure, connected to either a flat or round perforated internal tubing component (Fig. 9.6). This closed drainage system is commonly used in abdominal, breast, thoracic, and head and neck surgeries. The internal portion of the drain is placed in the surgical bed and may be trimmed to eliminate redundant tubing. A small incision in the skin, usually separate from the surgical incision, is used to allow the tubing to exit the body. Removing these drains may cause discomfort, as the interface between the perforated, collecting portion of the drain is larger than the drainage tube.

Blake

Blake drains are similar to JP drains, except they contain a continuous tube as opposed to a step off to the collecting portion of the tube. Additionally, instead of being perforated at the collecting portion of the tube, Blake drains contain external channels that allow fluid to be sucked into the drainage tube via capillary action and negative pressure (Fig. 9.7). The exiting portion of the tube is connected to a drainage bulb that when squeezed creates negative pressure. Pain is typically less severe when removing these drains as compared to that noted with JP drains.

Hemovac

Hemovac drains work in a similar fashion to JP and Blake drains. The difference in this type of drain is the collection reservoir itself. Shaped like an accordion that allows negative pressure to be created, the Hemovac drain is a closed, active drainage system (Fig. 9.8). The reservoir is much larger than a JP bulb and additionally has the potential for blood to be collected and given back to the patient as an autotransfusion.

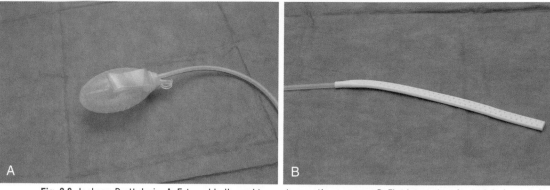

Fig. 9.6 Jackson-Pratt drain. A. External bulb used to create negative pressure. B. Flat internal perforated drainage tube.

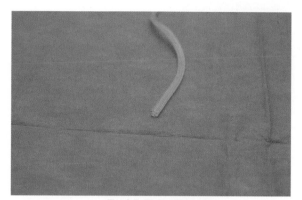

Fig. 9.7 Blake drain

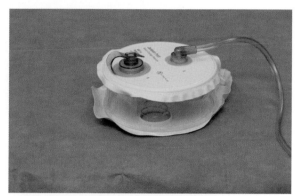

Fig. 9.8 Hemovac drain

Pigtail

Pigtail drains are smaller-caliber drains placed through the skin to drain a surgical site, abscess, or organ space. These drains are often placed under radiologic guidance by an interventional radiologist, although they may be inserted during surgical procedures as well. The curled end of a pigtail drain allows it to stay in place in the cavity in which it is placed and contains perforations for collecting fluid (Fig. 9.9). Pigtail drains are part of a closed drainage system and may be connected to either a negative pressure bulb, such as when draining an abscess or postoperative fluid, or a drainage bag, such as when used as cholecystostomy or nephrostomy tubes.

Sump

A sump drain (Salem sump drain) is a double-lumen drainage tube that creates an open, active drainage system. The inner lumen is connected to a drainage system and allows for active drainage of fluid from a surgical site. The outer lumen is open and allows air to replace the space where fluid was previously drained. This helps prevent clogging of the intake ports of the drain. One concern with this type of drain is the potential to introduce bacteria and other pathogens into the surgical site as air is

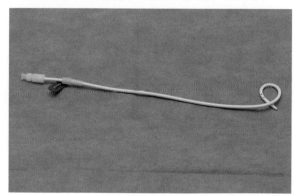

Fig. 9.9 Pigtail drain

introduced into the system. One of the most common examples of a sump drain is the nasogastric tube (discussed below).

Chest Tube

Chest tubes are comparatively larger drainage tubes inserted into the pleural space to form a closed drainage system (Fig. 9.10). They are commonly placed after thoracic surgery procedures and to drain a hemothorax, pleural effusion, or empyema, or evacuate a pneumothorax. Large fenestrations are present on the internal portion of the tube to drain fluid and air. These tend to

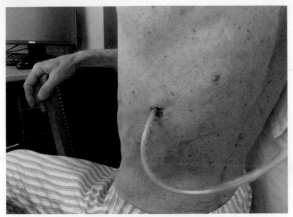

Fig. 9.10 Chest tube From Kuhajda I, Zarogoulidis K, Kougioumtzi I, et al. Tube thoracostomy; chest tube implantation and follow-up. *Journal of Thoracic Disease.* 2014;6(suppl 4):S470–S479.

be constructed of stiffer material to prevent them from collapsing during the respiratory process. Chest tubes are connected to a drainage canister that creates a constant low negative pressure to pull air and fluid from the pleural space without allowing it to reenter (Fig. 9.11).

Size of Drain

Each of the drains mentioned previously come in different sizes, varying based on their application. In general, the size of a drain should be chosen based on its intended use. For example, in children and confined surgical sites, smaller drains are more appropriate. Surgeries that necessitate postoperative drainage but have the potential for minimal blood loss and drainage (e.g., a laparoscopic pyeloplasty) may also be better served with smaller drains as opposed to larger ones.

Placing and Securing a Drain

Surgical drains should be placed adjacent to the site where fluid or potential fluid needs to be evacuated. Complicated cases may require multiple drains to adequately drain the surgical site. Although some surgeons will elect to place the drain through the main incision, surgical drains are more commonly placed at a separate site. In the case of open surgery, this usually requires a separate small incision to be made, whereas in the case of laparoscopic and robotic surgeries, the drain can be placed through one of the port sites. It is important to choose a port site that is small enough to not require fascial closure, as placing a drain and not doing so creates a risk of herniation, and closing the site around a drain risks breaking the closure suture as well as a weak fascial closure.

When creating a separate incision for a drain, a small stab wound should be made in the skin where the drain is to exit the body. Dissection through the remaining layers of tissue to enter the surgical site is performed. The surgical site itself dictates how to do so. For

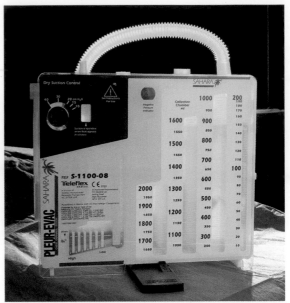

Fig. 9.11 Chest drainage canister. From Rothrock JC. Thoracic surgery. In: *Alexander's Care of the Patient in Surgery.* 14th ed. St. Louis, MO: Mosby; 2011:936–968.

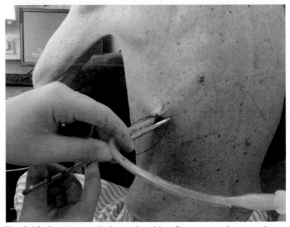

Fig. 9.12 Securing a drain to the skin after a procedure requires a suture to be placed through the skin and tied around the drain. From Kuhajda I, Zarogoulidis K, Kougioumtzi I, et al. Tube thoracostomy; chest tube implantation and follow-up. *Journal of Thoracic Disease.* 2014;6(suppl 4):S470–S479.

example, when placing a drain in the abdomen, a semi-sharp grasping instrument (e.g., a Kelly clamp or tonsil clamp) is placed through the stab wound and pushed through the remaining layers of tissue. The Kelly clamp then grasps the outside of the drain and is withdrawn to bring the drain to the outside.

Each surgical site additionally dictates how the drain should be secured to the patient. Larger drains, such as chest tubes, Hemovac drains, sump drains, JP drains, and Blake drains, often require a suture to be placed through the skin and around the drain to secure it in place (Fig. 9.12). Surgeon preference often

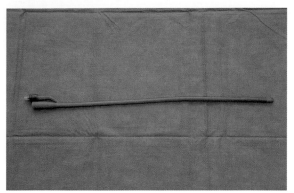

Fig. 9.13 Foley catheter

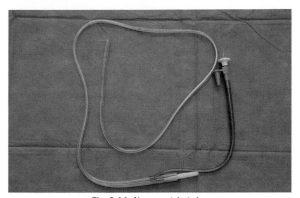

Fig. 9.14 Nasogastric tube

dictates the material and size of the suture. Monofilament sutures have less of a tendency to create an irritative skin reaction. The use of absorbable or nonabsorbable material is dictated by the length of time a drain may be needed. Some smaller drains in more delicate areas can be secured with adhesive or locking attachments that stick to the skin. This is particularly relevant for drains that allow for internal fixation, such as pigtail drains.

Foley Catheter

A Foley catheter (Fig. 9.13) is a tube placed through the urethra to collect urine. It is usually placed at the beginning of a procedure that has the potential to last for several hours, when ambulation will be limited postoperatively, when strict measurement of urine output is necessary, and following surgery on the lower urinary tract. Catheters come in a variety of diameters, tip shapes, and materials. Each application may mandate a certain type of catheter; however, the most commonly used are 16 or 18 French (F) in size. French measurement is equivalent to three times the diameter in millimeters, such that an 18F catheter is 6 mm in diameter. Catheters are kept in place by a balloon filled with water that is filled via a one-way valve adjacent to where the urine drains from the catheter. The balloon keeps the catheter from falling out by being too large to come out through the urethra. Catheters have recommended filling volumes written on the port of the catheter itself, most commonly 10 cc or 30 cc. Catheter-associated urinary tract infections (CAUTIs) have become increasingly prevalent, often with multidrug resistant bacteria, and are directly correlated with the length of time that they are left indwelling. It is therefore important to assess the need for a catheter postoperatively and to remove the catheter as early as possible.

Nasogastric Tube

Nasogastric (NG) tubes (Fig. 9.14) may be placed for surgeries that involve entry into the gastrointestinal (GI)

tract, bowel resection, or concern for postoperative ileus. As their name implies, they are placed through one of the nostrils and advanced into the stomach. They are usually hooked up to an intermittent suction device that pulls gastric contents out. There is usually a blue port that runs adjacent to the suction part that is open to the air. When suction is applied, it allows a small amount of air to enter the stomach to prevent the tube from sucking directly on the gastric wall. Their use removes and further prevents the buildup of gastric contents in the stomach and hence the rest of the digestive system. NG tubes continue to suction gastric contents from the stomach until they are removed, typically after return of bowel function.

SUTURING

Once the surgical site is inspected, hemostasis is achieved, and drains are placed, it is time to reconstruct the layers of the incision. Wound strength and minimizing risk of infection is dictated by the quality of wound closure. Even at its best, wound strength only approaches 80 to 90% of preprocedure strength.[15]

Different tissues provide different levels of strength to a surgical wound closure. For instance, the abdominal fascia provides nearly all of the closure strength for abdominal incisions, whereas the peritoneum provides nearly no closure strength.[15,16] Additionally, different areas of skin are subject to greater degrees of tension created by motion of underlying muscle. Incisions across joints on hands and feet are under greater force than areas such as the genitalia and face. The following review discusses the principles of abdominal wound closure by layer.

Peritoneum

The abdominal peritoneum is the innermost layer of an abdominal wound. This layer provides no strength to the overall closure, and therefore many surgeons will forego closure of the peritoneal layer. Additionally, numerous studies have demonstrated that the peritoneum reepithelializes by 48 to 72 hours.[17,18] It is, however, the layer in direct contact with the abdominal viscera, and therefore some surgeons choose to close it for two reasons: (1) during fascial closure, it prevents bowel from herniating through the wound and thus helps to prevent bowel injury during closure of the rest of the wound, and (2) in the event that wound dehiscence does occur, a closed peritoneal layer prevents evisceration.

When closure of the peritoneum is performed, care should be taken to avoid injury to the bowel and to ensure incorporation of only the peritoneal layer into the closure. A rapidly absorbing suture material such as Vicryl or chromic is typically chosen, and in most cases a size of 3-0 is more than sufficient. It is customary to perform a running closure of the peritoneum without placing tension on the suture as the closure is being performed.

Muscle

Muscle is a delicate tissue that will bleed and tear easily when too much force is placed on it. Moreover, if gathered and tied tightly, suture can strangulate the tissue. As such, if actual muscle tissue is brought together, it is approximated loosely. When a muscle is cut transversely during the course of a surgery, attempts to reapproximate the two cut ends of the muscle should be made. This is usually done by incorporating fascia in the repair, as suture can easily pull through the muscle. This facilitates healing and reduces loss of muscle strength postoperatively. When muscle is split, as is commonly done to the rectus muscles along the linea alba during midline abdominal surgeries, it is not necessary to reapproximate the split muscle. However, some surgeons will elect to do so to restore the anatomic relationship of the surgical wound. To reapproximate muscle, an absorbable suture such as chromic gut should be used. This suture is usually no larger than 2-0, and is more commonly 3-0, and the muscle is closed in an interrupted fashion with large spaces permissible in between sutures.

Fascia

Fascia is the connective tissue layer that attaches to and stabilizes muscle, separates the body into different compartments, and provides strength to prevent herniation of internal organs. As discussed, it is principally involved in providing strength to an incision after a surgical procedure. For this reason, it is imperative to ensure that an adequate fascial closure has been performed during incision closure.

The edges of the abdominal fascia should be reapproximated. In areas where two fascial layers overlap, such as in the flank, each layer is usually closed separately. The fascia may be closed with either a running continuous suture or in an interrupted fashion. The choice of a running continuous suture versus an

interrupted suture depends on both wound size and surgeon preference. Larger wounds may be more amenable to a running closure, whereas smaller wounds may be better closed with an interrupted technique. If performed as an interrupted closure, a figure-of-eight suturing technique may be chosen to allow for greater strength of each individual suture.

Regardless of technique, it is important to ensure that there are no significant gaps between sutures that would increase the risk of hernia formation. It is also important to make sure that there is not an excessive amount of tension placed on the suture material as it is being thrown. Doing so increases the risk that the suture will break. By convention, the suture should be thrown approximately 1 cm from the fascial edge. Increasing the distance from the fascial edge to greater than 1 cm increases the tension placed on the closure, increases the risk of ischemia, and increases the risk of hernia formation.[19] Placing sutures at a width of less than 1 cm from the incision places the closure at risk of tearing through the fascia and resultant hernia formation.

When performing closure of the fascia in adults, a delayed absorbing or nonabsorbable suture such as PDS is chosen. This is typically of a sufficient size, such as #0 or #1, to ensure adequate strength of the suture material. Alternatively, when smaller wounds that will not be subject to as much tension are closed, a Vicryl suture may be used. Again, usually a large-size suture is used, such as #0 or #1.

Subcutaneous Tissue

As with muscle, it is not always necessary to reapproximate the subcutaneous tissue during wound closure. In thin patients with minimal amounts of subcutaneous fat, for instance, attempting to close the subcutaneous tissue may distort the normal anatomy and make skin closure more difficult, thereby worsening the appearance of the surgical wound. In patients who are obese, it may be helpful to close the subcutaneous tissue to prevent seroma formation. Closing the subcutaneous layer prevents pockets of fluid, and potential infection, from developing underneath the skin. The subcutaneous layer should be closed with a 2-0 or 3-0 Vicryl or chromic suture. This layer is typically closed in an interrupted fashion by burying the suture, preventing the knot from causing pain and protruding through the incision. Because the goal is to reapproximate the tissue rather than fully closing the space, large gaps between sutures are permissible.

Skin

Skin closure is a part of most surgical procedures and can be accomplished in several ways. The choice of how to suture a skin incision depends on the length of the incision, the location, the tensile strength that the incision will be subject to postoperatively, and the patient's age.

Simple Suture

Skin suturing is a basic skill, and the reader should refer to Chapter 7 regarding the basics of suture placement. Interrupted simple sutures are the most commonly used method for closing skin, and are advantageous where higher tensile forces can disrupt the closure, such as in incisions across a joint or on the face. In areas subject to high degrees of force, a vertical mattress can be performed to increase closure strength. Simple running sutures are faster and may be used on areas of skin with favorable healing characteristics, such as the rugae of the scrotum. When a concern for wound infection exists, it may be advantageous to perform an interrupted skin closure so that small areas of the wound may be opened should an infection develop.

The choice of whether to use an absorbable or nonabsorbable suture material is based on clinical decision. When a high tensile area is being closed, a nonabsorbable suture is typically chosen to increase closure strength. When an absorbable suture material is chosen and the sutures will be allowed to dissolve without removal, chromic gut allows for a more rapidly dissolving suture.

Subcuticular Suture

Subcuticular sutures are performed for numerous types of surgical wounds. A running subcuticular suture (see Chapter 7) allows for no visible suture material to be seen outside the skin. Additionally, a dissolvable suture is used, foregoing the need to remove the suture in the future. This makes subcuticular suturing a favored method of closure for pediatric patients. Considering that no suture removal is required, performing a subcuticular suture closure eliminates postoperative pain from staples and nonabsorbable sutures. A 4-0 Monocryl, Biosyn, or Caprosyn suture is typically chosen for subcuticular skin closure. This suture technique places even tension along the length of the wound.

SKIN STAPLERS

Skin staples allow for an alternative form of closure compared to suturing. The main advantages of using staples include a shorter time to approximate the skin and the ability to open limited areas of the wound should a superficial infection develop. Disadvantages include increased postoperative pain as compared to sutures, especially upon removal. In stapling, an assistant uses tooth forceps to bring the skin edges together to hold them in place as the surgeon fires the

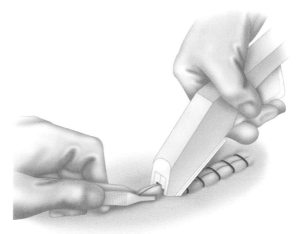

Fig. 9.15 Skin stapling is easily accomplished with an assistant who apposes the skin edges together.

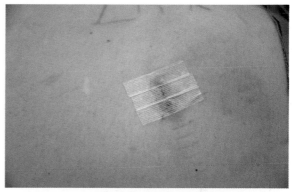

Fig. 9.16 Steri-Strips

stapler (Fig. 9.15). The cosmetic outcome of stapling skin for closure is no different from skin closed with sutures.[20]

DRESSINGS

Following skin closure, a sterile dressing is typically applied to the fresh wound. This protects the incision from mechanical abrasion from clothes or the environment and may help prevent infection. It can also collect blood and fluid that drains from the wound, as well as provide a more socially acceptable cosmetic appearance of the surgical site for the patient and family members. Dressings are typically left in place for 24 to 48 hours prior to being removed. Additionally, there are situations where no dressing may be applied at all.

Steri-Strips

Steri-Strips (Fig. 9.16) are thin pieces of reinforced adhesive that are placed across fresh wounds to take tension off the suture line. They are often used with a skin adhesive such as benzoin or Mastisol to provide stronger adherence. The most common use is across incisions that have been closed with a subcuticular suturing technique. Placing them across an incision allows additional tensile strength for incision closure. Steri-Strips usually stay in place until they begin falling off, typically weeks after being placed. It is important to place them over the incision and not pull the skin taut during placement, as this could result in blistering.

Covering the Incision

Multiple different types of dressings have been developed to cover a fresh surgical wound. In general, the dressing that provides acceptable protective properties while minimizing expense should be chosen. A simple dressing can consist of gauze secured by tape. There is no evidence that one dressing provides superior protection against infection compared to another; however, each situation may call for a specific dressing.[21] For example, for wounds in which a high degree of exudative drainage is expected, multiple gauze pads or an absorptive Army Battle Dressing (ABD) pads may be preferred (Fig. 9.17). In wounds where the gauze may stick to the incision site, a nonadherent material such as Telfa or Vaseline gauze may be used. Xeroform, alternatively, is a petrolatum-based dressing that is used to keep an incision moist and has antibacterial properties as well (Fig. 9.18). Hydrocolloid dressings are composed of biodegradable polymers meant to promote wound healing and are used primarily on area of skin breakdown, such as decubitus or venous stasis ulcers (Fig. 9.19). Foam dressing is applied to wick fluid away when a small or moderate amount of exudate is expected (Fig. 9.20).

Specialty Coverings
Wound Vacuum-Assisted Closure Systems

Negative pressure wound therapy, or wound vacuum-assisted closure (wound VAC) systems, are sealed systems that exert negative pressure over a wound. These systems use negative pressure to remove exudate from a wound and additionally increase circulation, bringing nutrients to a site of healing.

There are a variety of different forms of the device available. The standard wound VAC system uses foam placed in an open skin wound. This is covered by a protective dressing placed over the foam, which extends onto normal tissue (Fig. 9.21). This allows a seal to form and negative pressure to draw fluid from the wound. This allows healing to occur over time, decreasing the size of a wound and minimizing the risk of infection.

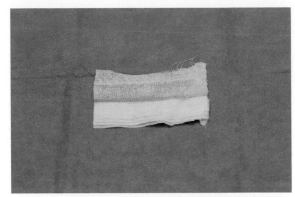

Fig. 9.18 Xeroform dressing material

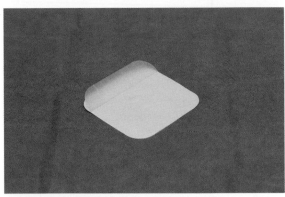

Fig. 9.19 Hydrocolloid dressing

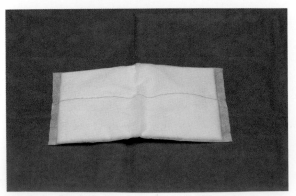

Fig. 9.17 Army Battle Dressing (ABD) pad

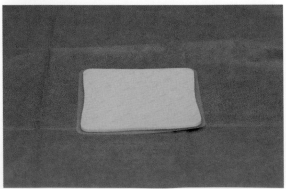

Fig. 9.20 Foam dressing

The Active Abdominal Therapy (ABThera) device is used for patients with an open abdomen. It is placed inside the open wound and allows for active removal of peritoneal fluid (Fig. 9.22). It also helps to protect the abdominal contents that would otherwise be open to the environment. ABThera VAC systems are required to be changed every few days.

The PREVENA incision management system is a disposable, battery-powered wound VAC device that is placed directly over closed surgical incisions (Fig. 9.23). It has been shown in multiple studies to decrease seroma formation, reduce the risk of postoperative SSI, and increase blood flow to surgical incisions.[22–24] Additionally, it allows excess exudative fluid to be continuously suctioned away from the wound. PREVENA VAC devices can be left in place for 2 to 7 days postoperatively.

Skin Glue

As an adjunct or alternative to skin closure with sutures, two forms of tissue adhesive are available. These two adhesives, n-2-butyl-cyanoacrylate (Histoacryl Blue, PeriAcryl) and 2-octyl-cyanoacrylate (DERMABOND, SurgiSeal), rapidly form a complete bond to the skin (usually within 3 minutes) and typically slough off within 5 to 10 days.[25] They form a protective antimicrobial barrier and allow the underlying tissue to heal normally. Skin adhesives are typically used on smaller incisions and optimally in areas that are not subject to a great deal of tension.

Tape

A variety of different types of tape and adhesives have been developed for medical use. Again, as with Steri-Strips, it is important to not place tape taut across the dressing, as this may lead to blistering of the skin. Paper tape is a mild adhesive that is often used to redress surgical wounds after removing the initial dressing (Fig. 9.24). It rarely causes adverse reactions that can sometimes occur with other types of adhesives. Because

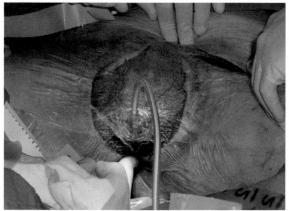

Fig. 9.21 Standard wound VAC system From Zagli G, Cianchi G, Degl'innocenti S, et al. Treatment of Fournier's gangrene with combination of vacuum-assisted closure therapy, hyperbaric oxygen therapy, and protective colostomy. *Case Reports in Anesthesiology.* 2011;2011:430983.

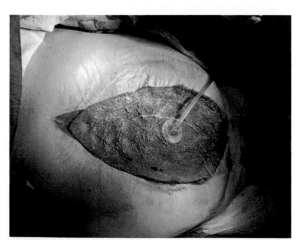

Fig. 9.22 Active Abdominal Therapy (ABThera) device From Wachal K, Krasinski Z, Szmyt K, Bialecki J, Slawek S, Oszkinis G. Acute pancreatitis complicated by rupture of abdominal aortic aneurysm. *Gastroenterology Review.* 2016;11(2):136–138.

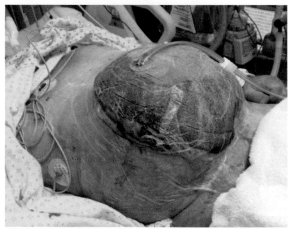

Fig. 9.23 PREVENA incision management system From Zuriarrain A, et al. The sentinel placement of an open abdomen negative pressure unit. *Int J Surg Case Rep.* 2011;2(1):4–5.

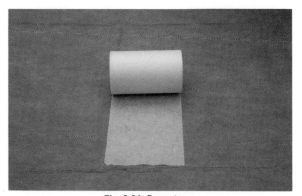

Fig. 9.24 Paper tape

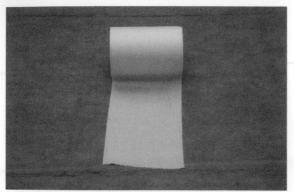

Fig. 9.25 Silk tape

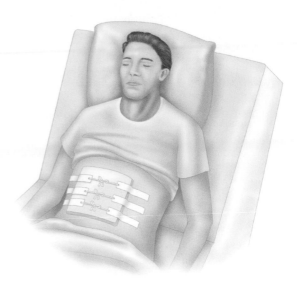

Fig. 9.27 Montgomery straps

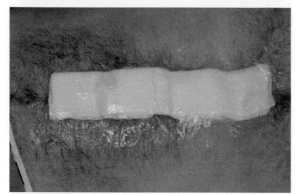

Fig. 9.26 Multiple pieces of Tegaderm used to adequately cover a long surgical wound

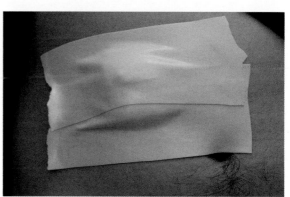

Fig. 9.28 Pressure dressing consisting of stretch tape covering multiple pieces of gauze

of its mild nature, it offers less adhesive strength than others. In general, paper tape dressings are not sterile. Silk tape, alternatively, is a strong adhesive that can be used to cover surgical wounds (Fig. 9.25). It is extremely useful when a wound is in an area of high tension where ordinary tape would fall off. Because of its strong adhesive properties, silk tape can tear skin when changing in some patients.

Tegaderm is a fixed-size, clear adhesive sheath that can be placed over a wound dressing. It comes in a sterile package and stretches easily to accommodate patient movement. Multiple pieces of Tegaderm can be overlapped to create a longer or wider strip of adhesive (Fig. 9.26). Tegaderm is commonly used to dress surgical wounds because of its pliable nature and impermeability to water and other fluids in the environment. In addition, clinicians are able to see the color and consistency of exudate on bandages underneath it. It also has less of a tendency to tear skin than other adhesive materials, such as silk tape. Tegaderm serves as an effective wound dressing but is more costly than other adhesive materials.

Montgomery straps (Fig. 9.27) are specialized wound dressings that allow for improved patient comfort when frequent wound dressing changes are required. These dressings consist of an adhesive strip that is placed on the body distant from the site of the wound. Connected to this adhesive strip is a nonadhesive strip and a tie. Placed across from another strip of material, the ties can be secured together to hold a dressing in place beneath it. Frequently, multiple straps are placed to secure a single dressing.

Pressure dressings, as their name implies, are special dressings designed to exert pressure on a wound. These dressings are typically used to promote hemostasis. Silk tape may be used to cover multiple pieces of gauze or other material, therefore exerting pressure on the wound; however, it is important to remember that silk tape drawn taut on skin may cause skin breakdown. Alternatively, stretch tape that is milder on skin may be used (Fig. 9.28). Video 9.1 demonstrates the most common methods of skin closure, including how to apply Steri-Strips and skin glue.

REFERENCES

1. Barnes S, Spencer M, Graham D, Johnson HB. Surgical wound irrigation: a call for evidence-based standardization of practice. *American Journal of Infection Control.* 2014;42(5):525–529.
2. Mueller TC, Loos M, Haller B, et al. Intra-operative wound irrigation to reduce surgical site infections after abdominal surgery: a systematic review and meta-analysis. *Langenbeck's Archives of Surgery.* 2015;400(2):167–181.
3. Hainge F, Bucholz JM. Principles and methods of clean surgical wound irrigation. *Journal of Foot Surgery.* 1982;21(4):241–246.
4. Mahomed K, Ibiebele I, Buchanan J. The Betadine trial—antiseptic wound irrigation prior to skin closure at caesarean section to prevent surgical site infection: a randomised controlled trial. *Australian and New Zealand Journal of Obstetrics and Gynaecology.* 2016;56(3):301–306.
5. Camp MA. Hemostatic agents: a guide to safe practice for perioperative nurses. *AORN Journal.* 2014;100(2):131–147.
6. Mannucci PM. Hemostatic drugs. *New England Journal of Medicine.* 1998;339(4):245–253.
7. Peralta E. Overview of topical hemostatic agents and tissues adhesives used in surgery. In: Sanfey H, ed. *UpToDate.* https://www.uptodate.com/contents/overview-of-topical-hemostatic-agents-and-tissues-adhesives
8. Hong YM, Loughlin KR. The use of hemostatic agents and sealants in urology. *Journal of Urology.* 2006;176(6 Pt 1):2367–2374.
9. Ereth MH, Schaff M, Ericson EF, Wetjen NM, Nuttall GA, Oliver Jr WC. Comparative safety and efficacy of topical hemostatic agents in a rat neurosurgical model. *Neurosurgery.* 2008;63(4 suppl 2):369–372; discussion 72.
10. Bak JB, Singh A, Shekarriz B. Use of gelatin matrix thrombin tissue sealant as an effective hemostatic agent during laparoscopic partial nephrectomy. *Journal of Urology.* 2004;171(2 Pt 1):780–782.
11. Uribe CA, Eichel L, Khonsari S, et al. What happens to hemostatic agents in contact with urine? An in vitro study. *Journal of Endourology.* 2005;19(3):312–317.
12. Spotnitz WD, Burks S. Hemostats, sealants, and adhesives: components of the surgical toolbox. *Transfusion.* 2008;48(7):1502–1516.
13. Chao HH, Torchiana DF. BioGlue: albumin/glutaraldehyde sealant in cardiac surgery. *Journal of Cardiac Surgery.* 2003;18(6):500–503.
14. Pursifull NF, Morey AF. Tissue glues and nonsuturing techniques. *Current Opinion in Urology.* 2007;17(6):396–401.
15. Mizell J. Principles of abdominal wall closure. In: Sanfey H, ed. *UpToDate.* https://www.uptodate.com/contents/principles-of-abdominal-wall-closure
16. Douglas DM. The healing of aponeurotic incisions. *British Journal of Surgery.* 1952;40(159):79–84.
17. Gurusamy KS, Cassar Delia E, Davidson BR. Peritoneal closure versus no peritoneal closure for patients undergoing non-obstetric abdominal operations. *Cochrane Database of Systematic Reviews.* 2013;(7):CD010424.
18. Tulandi T, Al-Jaroudi D. Nonclosure of peritoneum: a reappraisal. *American Journal of Obstetrics and Gynecology.* 2003;189(2):609–612.
19. Millbourn D, Cengiz Y, Israelsson LA. Effect of stitch length on wound complications after closure of midline incisions: a randomized controlled trial. *Archives of Surgery.* 2009;144(11):1056–1059.
20. Iavazzo C, Gkegkes ID, Vouloumanou EK, Mamais I, Peppas G, Falagas ME. Sutures versus staples for the management of surgical wounds: a meta-analysis of randomized controlled trials. *American Surgeon.* 2011;77(9):1206–1221.
21. Dumville JC, Gray TA, Walter CJ, Sharp CA, Page T. Dressings for the prevention of surgical site infection. *Cochrane Database of Systematic Reviews.* 2014;(9):CD003091.
22. Blackham AU, Farrah JP, McCoy TP, Schmidt BS, Shen P. Prevention of surgical site infections in high-risk patients with laparotomy incisions using negative-pressure therapy. *American Journal of Surgery.* 2013;205(6):647–654.
23. Bonds AM, Novick TK, Dietert JB, Araghizadeh FY, Olson CH. Incisional negative pressure wound therapy significantly reduces surgical site infection in open colorectal surgery. *Diseases of the Colon and Rectum.* 2013;56(12):1403–1408.
24. Pachowsky M, Gusinde J, Klein A, et al. Negative pressure wound therapy to prevent seromas and treat surgical incisions after total hip arthroplasty. *International Orthopaedics.* 2012;36(4):719–722.
25. Singer AJ, Quinn JV, Hollander JE. The cyanoacrylate topical skin adhesives. *American Journal of Emergency Medicine.* 2008;26(4):490–496.

CHAPTER 10

POSTOPERATIVE CARE

At the completion of a surgical procedure, the patient is placed on a stretcher and brought to the recovery area, where postoperative care commences. The postoperative period can be divided into three stages, each with their own considerations: immediate recovery, time on the surgical ward, and at-home convalescence. Each is part of a continuum, with details regarding care and goals to ensure optimal recovery and outcomes dependent on the specific surgery performed.

At the conclusion of surgery, the circulating nurse contacts the recovery area to secure a spot for the patient and communicate pertinent details. Information such as the type of surgery, blood loss, fluids, number of intravenous (IV) lines, drains, and general patient condition is relayed. The physician team writes postoperative orders for the nursing staff to follow, addressing diet, activity, medications, deep venous thrombosis (DVT) prophylaxis, dressing care, monitoring, laboratory testing, and fluid management. Once the patient arrives in the recovery room, vital signs are obtained and the patient is assessed for pain, arousability, integrity of dressings, respiratory status, and hemodynamic stability. The nursing staff's role is to pick up on critical acute issues, such as bleeding, and start setting up baseline pain control. Any issues are addressed, and once the nursing staff determine a patient is relatively comfortable and stable, the patient is ready to be transferred to the floor, specialized unit, or even discharged home. Once again, communication with the receiving unit is important to ensure smooth patient progress. On the floor, focus transitions to the patient regaining basic activity such as gastrointestinal (GI) function, ambulation, and self-reliance. Once a patient is deemed safe to be in his own home or another facility with a higher level of care, such as a rehabilitation facility, he is discharged with specific instructions aimed at facilitating continued recovery.

DIET

Patients undergoing ambulatory surgical procedures typically may resume their normal preprocedure diet within a few hours following the procedure. In the case of patients undergoing minor procedures that do not pose a significant risk for postoperative ileus, the greatest consideration for diet advancement is anesthesia duration and adverse reactions. Many patients report feeling nauseated after undergoing anesthesia, and therefore oral intake of food and liquids should be delayed until this period has passed. Postoperative nausea and vomiting (PONV) is positively correlated with the duration of anesthesia, female gender, surgeries that involve the head and neck or abdomen, and a history of PONV.[1,2]

To reduce the effects of anesthesia on PONV, medications such as selective serotonin receptor antagonists (including ondansetron, granisetron, ramosetron, dolasetron, and tropisetron), metoclopramide, and dexamethasone can help.[3] Table 10.1 presents a review of commonly used antiemetic medications for PONV. The combination of two drugs can provide an additive effect.[4] These medications may be administered preventatively at the end of a procedure. Alternatively, medications may be given as needed.

After reversal of anesthesia in patients undergoing ambulatory surgical procedures, it is important to confirm that they can tolerate oral intake prior to discharge. Patients should be assessed to ensure that they are sufficiently awake to avoid aspiration of liquids and food. After awakening, a trial of liquids is usually initiated prior to moving to solid foods. When patients have tolerated food in the recovery room, and after meeting other postoperative criteria for discharge, they can be safely discharged from the ambulatory surgical center.

In patients who have undergone procedures requiring hospital admission but not involving the GI tract, entry into the abdomen, or certain head and neck procedures, diet advancement typically occurs rapidly. Procedures of prolonged duration that satisfy the preceding criteria may benefit from a greater period of diet restriction for adequate control of PONV and anesthesia reversal, but in general there is no contraindication to advancing the diet to regular food. As in patients undergoing ambulatory surgical procedures, oral intake is often advanced rapidly from liquids to solid food.

In patients undergoing procedures that involve entry into the abdomen but not involving the

Table 10.1 Antiemetic Medications for Postoperative Nausea and Vomiting

Medication	Nausea RR (95% CI)	Vomiting RR (95% CI)	Nausea or Vomiting RR (95% CI)	Rescue Antiemetic RR (95% CI)
Cyclizine	0.65 (0.47–0.90)	0.57 (0.43–0.75)	0.68 (0.58–0.80)	0.27 (0.14–0.62)
Dexamethasone	0.57 (0.48–0.69)	0.51 (0.46–0.57)	0.49 (0.44–0.54)	0.50 (0.42–0.59)
Dolasetron	0.82 (0.76–0.90)	0.63 (0.51–0.76)	0.72 (0.62–0.83)	0.67 (0.57–0.79)
Droperidol	0.65 (0.60–0.71)	0.65 (0.61–0.70)	0.62 (0.58–0.67)	0.53 (0.47–0.60)
Granisetron	0.53 (0.45–0.63)	0.40 (0.35–0.46)	0.39 (0.31–0.48)	0.29 (0.22–0.39)
Metoclopramide	0.82 (0.76–0.88)	0.75 (0.70–0.81)	0.76 (0.70–0.82)	0.78 (0.69–0.88)
Ondansetron	0.68 (0.63–0.74)	0.55 (0.50–0.59)	0.56 (0.50–0.63)	0.55 (0.49–0.61)
Prochlorperazine	0.73 (0.56–0.96)	0.68 (0.52–0.89)	0.68 (0.55–0.86)	0.49 (0.22–1.08)
Ramosetron	0.62 (0.40–0.96)	0.42 (0.28–0.63)	0.51 (0.39–0.68)	0.38 (0.15–0.99)
Tropisetron	0.77 (0.71–0.84)	0.59 (0.50–0.69)	0.70 (0.61–0.81)	0.62 (0.53–0.72)

Modified from Carlisle JB, Stevenson CA. Drugs for preventing postoperative nausea and vomiting. Cochrane Database of Systematic Reviews. 2006(3):CD004125.

GI tract, surgeon preference may dictate how the patient's diet is advanced. Patients who report significant PONV may benefit from restriction to a liquid diet or no oral intake (NPO) until PONV subsides. Open abdominal procedures often result in a greater period of postoperative ileus than laparoscopic and robotic procedures, and therefore patients may benefit from a period of NPO until the return of GI function. This decision is often based on surgeon preference, the complexity of the surgery, and the time under anesthesia.

Laparoscopic and robotic minimally invasive surgeries may allow for earlier return of GI function and reduced PONV, thereby allowing diet advancement more rapidly than following open abdominal procedures. Whereas the dogma for open surgical procedures has shifted from immediate NPO to a liquid diet for many intra-abdominal procedures, minimally invasive procedures have seen a similar shift from liquid to solid oral intake in the immediate postoperative period.

Abdominal procedures that involve entry into the GI tract include small or large bowel resections, gastrectomy, esophagectomy, gastric bypass, or ileal substitution procedures such as the creation of an ileal conduit or ileal ureter. Many of these procedures may require a prolonged period of NPO. Again, whereas the dogma has begun to shift to allow the earlier introduction of liquids, and to some extent solid foods, in these patients most surgeons elect to keep a patient NPO until the return of GI function after a major abdominal procedure that involves entry into the GI tract. This is due to the prolonged ileus that these patients typically experience, the concern for disrupting a newly created GI tract anastomosis, and sometimes profound PONV. In these patients, some surgeons also elect to place a nasogastric tube (NGT) at the time of surgery to further reduce GI tract contents. In

most cases, after return of flatus, the diet is typically advanced to liquids only, followed by advancement to a regular diet after the patient has a bowel movement. Many variations on the way a patient's diet is advanced are possible, and they are often dictated by surgeon preference.

In patients who are kept NPO for a prolonged period of time, alternative methods of providing nutrition should be considered. Typically, a week to 10 days of starvation is considered acceptable when administering IV fluids, although instituting alternative methods of nutrition earlier may result in improved wound healing and surgical outcomes. This may include any number of measures, including delivery of enteral nutrition via NGT or nasojejunal feeding tube (Fig. 10.1), or placement of a jejunostomy feeding tube when a greater period of NPO is expected. In patients for whom the delivery of enteral nutrition is contraindicated, consideration should be given for total parenteral nutrition (TPN), which involves administering sugars, lipids, protein, vitamins, minerals, and other nutrients via IV administration. TPN is most commonly used in patients with GI malabsorptive disorders or in patients with GI tract fistulas. TPN may also be used in patients who are intubated or are in a coma, although enteral feeding is preferred in these patients. Additionally, giving TPN requires the placement of a peripherally inserted central catheter (PICC) line for administration.

Additional consideration should be given for nutritional supplements in patients who are nutritionally deprived. This typically includes patients who are elderly and those with decreased caloric intake. Supplements include Ensure, Boost, and Glucerna, as well as Nepro shakes for patients with renal impairment (Fig. 10.2). Adequate caloric and nutritional intake in postoperative patients aids in wound healing and a sense of well-being, and has been shown to decrease infectious complications and reduce the length of hospital stay.[5]

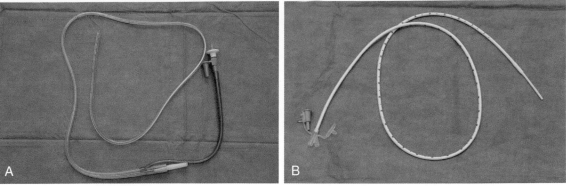

Fig. 10.1 Enteral feeding tubes. A. Nasogastric tube. B. Nasojejunal feeding tube.

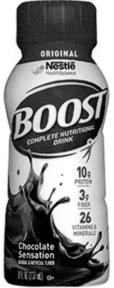

Fig. 10.2 Boost nutritional supplement shake. From https://www.boost.com/products

ANALGESIA

Postoperative pain control is a significant consideration for patients undergoing surgical procedures. The main goals of providing postoperative pain control are to reduce patient distress, increase mobility, reduce length of hospital stay, and improve patient satisfaction. Inadequate postoperative pain control may increase complications and delay recovery from surgery. Pain is the most-feared side effect following surgery for many patients. It is crucial to get pain managed properly to allow patients to progress with other aspects of healing. Pain is quantitated via validated scales, usually ranging from 1 to 10, with 10 being the worst pain of one's life. An important principle of pain control is to try and avoid a patient from reaching severe pain, as it is more difficult to manage than through maintenance regimens of pain control. As such, pain medication should be offered and available throughout the recovery period.

However, as the side effects from pain medications can impede healing (e.g., ileus, confusion), it is important not to overmedicate patients. This balance is individual to each patient.

Different procedures result in varying amounts of pain and will therefore require different modalities of analgesic delivery. These primarily include oral, IV, and epidural delivery but may also incorporate transdermal administration. Pain medication can primarily be classified as a nonsteroidal anti-inflammatory drug (NSAID) or an opioid medication but can also include acetaminophen (Table 10.2).[6,7]

NSAIDs are increasingly being used for postoperative pain control. They work by blocking the enzyme cyclooxygenase, thereby decreasing production of prostaglandins. This decrease in the level of prostaglandins, which usually mediate nociception, results in the sensation of reduced pain. NSAID use has been found to adequately control pain for surgeries resulting in minor to moderate degrees of pain while reducing some of the complications associated with opioid pain medications. NSAIDs rarely result in mental confusion or GI disturbances, including constipation and PONV, which can be associated with opioid medications. Additionally, the use of NSAIDs has been found to result in a decreased use of opioid analgesics.[8] NSAIDs are usually given via oral administration, although the use of IV ketorolac (Toradol) has recently grown in popularity owing to its superb pain control.

Opioids are the mainstay of postoperative pain control in both the immediate postoperative period and for prolonged pain control. Multiple different routes of delivery exist for opioid pain medications, including oral, IV, transdermal, and neuraxial (epidural) routes of delivery. Their mechanism of action for pain control occurs at the level of the dorsal root ganglia and in the cerebral cortex. Several adverse side effects also occur with opioid medications owing to their cross actions on the central nervous system

Table 10.2 Common Medications Used for Perioperative Pain Control

Drug	Method of Administration	Usual Dose
Opioids		
Codeine	PO, immediate release	30–60 mg q4–6 hours
Fentanyl	IV	25–50 mcg q1–2 hours
	Transdermal patch	12–25 mcg q72 hours
Hydrocodone	PO, immediate release	5–10 mg q6 hours
	PO, extended release	10–20 mg q12–24 hours
Hydromorphone	IV	0.3–1 mg q2–4 hours
	PO, immediate release	2–4 mg q3–4 hours
Morphine	IV	2–5 mg q2–4 hours
	PO, immediate release	10–30 mg q4 hours
	PO, controlled release	15 mg BID
Oxycodone	PO, immediate release	5–15 mg q4–6 hours
	PO, controlled release	10 mg BID
NSAIDs		
Ibuprofen	PO	400 mg q4–6 hours
Ketorolac	IV	15–30 mg q6 hours
	PO	10 mg q4–6 hours
Aspirin	PO	325–650 mg q4–6 hours
Naproxen	PO	250–500 mg q12 hours
Diclofenac	PO	50 mg q8 hours
Acetaminophen	PO, immediate release	325–650 mg q4–6 hours
	IV	1000 mg q6 hours

PO, by mouth; IV, intravenous; BID, twice a day; NSAIDs, nonsteroidal anti-inflammatory drugs. Modified from Mariano E. Management of acute perioperative pain. In: Fanciullo G, ed. UpTo-Date. http://www.uptodate.com/contents/management-of-acute-perioperative-pain; Solomon D. NSAIDs: therapeutic use and variability of response in adults. In: Furst D, ed. UpToDate. http://www.uptodate.com/contents/nsaids-therapeutic-use-and-variability-of-response-in-adults

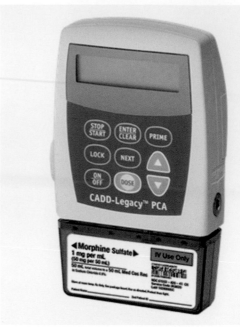

Fig. 10.3 Patient-controlled analgesia (PCA) device. From Smiths Medical. Available at https://www.smiths-medical.com/products

(CNS) and bowel, including mental confusion, sedation, respiratory suppression, constipation, nausea, and vomiting.

Opioid medications are often given in combination with acetaminophen or ibuprofen when delivered via the oral route. This allows for a reduction in opioid side effects while combining two different pain medications with differing mechanisms of action. These medications are particularly effective in postoperative patients requiring pain control after discharge from the hospital.

In more acute postoperative patients with greater levels of pain, opioids can be delivered via IV administration, either as an IV push or through a patient-controlled analgesia (PCA) device (Fig. 10.3). IV pushes of pain medication have the advantage of a more rapid onset of action than medications delivered via the oral route, although they tend to have a shorter duration of action. PCA devices can be programmed to deliver a basal amount of pain medication over time and also allow for on-demand dosing controlled by patients. Patient-controlled delivery of pain medication is usually programmed with a lockout period to prevent overdosing, during which additional pushes of the PCA button will not deliver more pain medication.

Epidural delivery of opioid medications is an extremely effective method of providing postoperative pain control. Via use of an epidural catheter and delivery of pain medication, procedures that would otherwise result in a significant amount of pain are greatly improved. Epidural catheters are usually placed prior to induction of anesthesia and often remain indwelling for 3 to 4 days postoperatively. Like PCAs, they allow for a continuous delivery of pain medication, albeit to the epidural space as opposed to IV administration. Additionally, they can allow for on-demand dosing through patient-controlled epidural analgesia (PCEA) buttons (Fig. 10.4). Because they are delivered to the epidural space as opposed to oral or IV administration, they also have the advantage of decreasing CNS and GI adverse side effects.

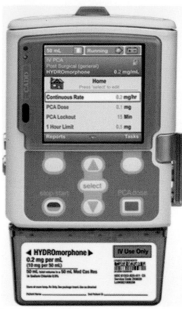

Fig. 10.4 Patient-controlled epidural analgesia (PCEA) device. From Smiths Medical. Available at https://www.smiths-medical.com/products

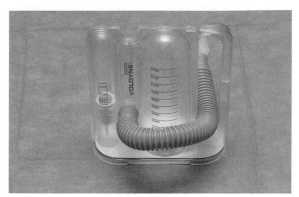

Fig. 10.5 Incentive spirometer

Once an epidural catheter is removed, patients are typically transitioned to either IV or oral pain medications for ongoing analgesia.

PULMONARY CONSIDERATIONS

Postoperative pulmonary complications can be some of the most devastating yet preventable causes of postoperative morbidity. Atelectasis, pneumonia, pulmonary embolism, aspiration, and pulmonary edema are some of the most frequent causes of morbidity in postsurgical patients. In fact, it is estimated that pulmonary complications can occur in up to 70% of patients undergoing upper abdominal surgeries.[9] For this reason, several measures should be taken to ensure an optimal pulmonary outcome in the postoperative period.

The first step in preventing postoperative pulmonary complications is to optimize pulmonary function preoperatively. This includes smoking cessation, achieving adequate exercise tolerance, and optimization of comorbidities such as chronic obstructive pulmonary disease (COPD) and asthma. Postoperatively, pain control prevents splinting and pain when breathing, allowing patients to take a deep breath and exert maximal respiratory effort. It also allows patients to ambulate more easily, allowing them to regain strength and prevent the development of DVT.

Lung expansion techniques, including deep breathing exercises and incentive spirometry, decrease pulmonary complications in the postoperative period. These techniques have been shown to prevent pulmonary complications such as atelectasis and pneumonia from developing.[10] Most incentive spirometers, such as the one in Fig. 10.5, have two separate indicator gauges. The larger gauge reveals the inspiratory volume of a breath. The smaller, secondary gauge reveals the velocity at which air is inspired and is usually described on a Likert scale of "Good," "Better," and "Best." To use an incentive spirometer, a patient should place the mouthpiece in her mouth and hold the device so that the two gauges can be seen. The patient takes a slow, sustained deep breath in, holding it for a few seconds at the end of inspiration. This process should be repeated multiple times per hour. The use of an incentive spirometer maintains optimal lung volumes and prevents atelectasis and pneumonia by keeping alveoli open.

Patients with preoperative comorbidities deserve special consideration in the postoperative period. Patients with COPD should be optimized prior to undergoing surgery and should also be maintained on their regimen of bronchodilators and inhaled corticosteroids postoperatively. Systemic corticosteroids may impair wound healing and should be tapered preoperatively, if possible. Additionally, because of the significant stress that surgery places on these patients, consultation with a pulmonologist is warranted.

Patients with asthma should continue their home regimen of corticosteroids and bronchodilators in the postoperative period. Asthma tends to manifest as episodic wheezing that is relieved with bronchodilators. In reliable patients, it is advisable to allow them free access to an inhaler at the bedside for when they experience symptoms of asthma. As pulmonary edema may manifest similarly to an asthma attack, it is important to consider this in the differential diagnosis when patients are undergoing IV fluid hydration, especially when symptoms do not improve with normal rescue measures, such as bronchodilator inhalers and albuterol nebulizers. To this end, it is also important in all postoperative patients to avoid excessive hydration, which could lead to pulmonary edema, but especially those at risk for pulmonary edema, such as patients with congestive heart failure. Moreover, patients on chronic diuretic therapy may need continued postoperative diuresis to remove fluid and avoid an exacerbation of pulmonary edema or congestive heart failure.

AMBULATION

Early ambulation is a critical component of the postoperative recovery plan for surgical patients. Individuals who are out of bed and ambulating earlier tend to have a quicker and more efficient recovery. Other than patients who were nonambulatory prior to surgery or patients in whom ambulation is contraindicated immediately after their procedure, as is the case with some orthopedic surgical procedures, most patients should be out of bed and ambulating no later than postoperative day 1.

Numerous studies have demonstrated the positive impact of ambulation on postoperative recovery. These benefits include a shorter length of hospital stay, lower hospital costs, and improved pain control, as well as a decrease in complications such as atelectasis, pneumonia, and DVT. Even in those patients who have developed a DVT, ambulation is not contraindicated. In fact, patients with a confirmed DVT do not experience a higher incidence of pulmonary embolism as compared to patients on bed rest but instead do experience a decrease in their level of pain.[11]

Of the most consistent and notable effects of early ambulation is a decreased length of hospital stay.[12-14] Even patients who are out of bed as little as 1 day sooner than their nonambulatory peers tend to be discharged from the hospital with a shorter length of stay. Additionally, in patients undergoing orthopedic hip and knee replacement surgeries, early ambulation has been associated with improved joint function and a decreased need for discharge to a high-level care facility.[13,14] Conversely, patients with a delay in getting out of bed have been found to have poorer overall function at 2 months postoperatively and greater mortality at 6 months.[15] These results definitively argue for early ambulation in patients after surgery.

Whereas it may be difficult for some patients to ambulate at their baseline level in the immediate postoperative period, a laudable goal for these patients is to steadily increase their daily amount of walking. All patients should be out of bed and to a chair as early as possible, followed by ambulation soon thereafter. This is typically done on postoperative day 1 for most major procedures, although some patients may be able to sit in a chair on the same day as the surgery. For patients who consistently have difficulty with ambulation, or in whom ambulation was difficult prior to

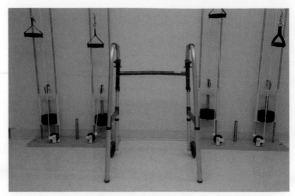

Fig. 10.6 Rolling walker

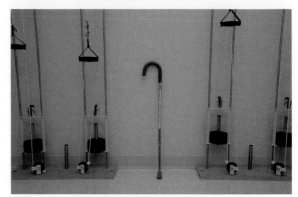

Fig. 10.7 Walking cane

surgery, physical therapy with a structured program of ambulation is beneficial. Multiple devices and aids are available to help patients reach the goal of ambulation. Rolling walkers allow patients to support their weight with their arms, relieving some of the effort of ambulation (Fig. 10.6). Alternatively, crutches or a cane may help patients support the weight of one lower extremity (Fig. 10.7). These assistive devices are useful in patients requiring less support than that provided by a rolling walker or in patients who need to minimize weight bearing on one lower extremity.

DVT PROPHYLAXIS

A DVT in the postoperative period can be devastating to a patient's recovery. As one of the most common and preventable complications after surgery, the healthcare team and patients alike must work together to prevent this potentially fatal complication. The type of DVT prophylaxis administered postoperatively is largely driven by preoperative patient characteristics, as well as the surgical procedure and intraoperative findings.

For a detailed discussion of the causes of DVT and categorization of patients into very low risk, low risk, moderate risk, or high risk for development of DVT, refer to Chapter 4. As venous stasis remains one of the leading contributors to the development of DVT, the foremost prevention is early ambulation, as it promotes blood return from the lower extremities.

In addition to early ambulation, other modalities are available for the prevention of DVT in surgical patients. These include mechanical prophylaxis such as intermittent pneumatic compression (IPC), subcutaneous low-dose unfractionated heparin (SQH or HSQ), and subcutaneous low-molecular-weight heparin (LMWH). The American College of Chest Physicians provides specific recommendations for the prevention of DVT and pulmonary embolism in surgical patients.[16] Although the full extent of these recommendations, including considerations for prophylaxis after various types of surgical procedures, is outside the scope of this text, general recommendations for prophylaxis are outlined in the following.

Patients at low risk for the development of DVT after surgery should preferably undergo mechanical prophylaxis over no DVT prophylaxis at all. This includes the use of IPC at all times when in bed and preferably when in a chair. After hospital discharge, continued ambulation is recommended for sustained DVT prevention. Patients at moderate risk for the development of DVT should undergo prophylaxis with either LMWH, SQH, or mechanical prophylaxis. Although not explicitly stated in the guidelines, many surgeons will use both mechanical prophylaxis and pharmacologic prophylaxis for preventing DVT in these patients. High-risk patients, alternatively, should receive combined mechanical and pharmacologic DVT prophylaxis. Additionally, in patients at high risk for the development of DVT in whom surgery was performed for cancer, extending the duration of pharmacologic prophylaxis with LMWH for a total of 4 weeks after surgery should be considered.

WOUND CARE

Proper care of surgical wounds is important to prevent surgical site infection (SSI) and promote wound healing. Different surgical wounds will require different types of dressings and provider involvement for ongoing care. For most closed surgical wounds, the original sterilely placed dressing should be left in place for 24 to 48 hours following surgery. This allows for adequate skin epithelialization to occur and minimizes the risk of concomitant infection. Most closed surgical wounds will require little more than periodic wound inspection for signs of infection. For closed surgical wounds in which the original dressing is clean, additional dressing of the wound is typically unnecessary. For those wounds that continue to produce exudate, the wound may be covered with a clean dressing to prevent soiling of the patient's clothes and bedding material. In most cases, placing a piece of clean gauze over the wound and covering it with a nonirritating adhesive, such as paper tape, is sufficient. This dressing can be changed as necessary and removed when leakage ceases.

Steri-Strips aid in wound closure by allowing an additional strength measure to keep the edges of a wound together. They are often placed over wounds closed with a running subcuticular suture and should be allowed to stay in place until the time at which they fall off. This typically occurs between 2 and 4 weeks after surgery. Until that time, patients may bathe (unless otherwise prohibited by the type of surgery that was performed) and should be instructed to dab over the surgical wound as opposed to vigorously scrubbing.

Staples and nonabsorbable sutures are typically removed between 7 and 14 days after surgery, depending on the surgical site and progress of healing. Special suture removal kits (Fig. 10.8) and staple removers (Fig. 10.9) are often used for this purpose. After staple or suture removal, Steri-Strips may be placed over the surgical wound for continued support. Steri-Strips should also be allowed to spontaneously fall off.

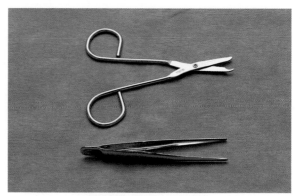

Fig. 10.8 Suture removal kit

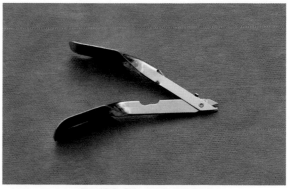

Fig. 10.9 Skin staple remover

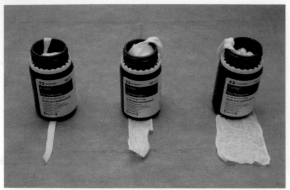

Fig. 10.10 Packing material for ongoing wound care; 1/4-inch, 1-inch, and 2-inch widths

Many surgical procedures performed because of infection (e.g., superficial abscesses and Fournier's gangrene) will require the wound to remain open postoperatively to prevent persistent infection. These wounds may be allowed to close spontaneously, may be surgically closed at some point in the future, or may require special grafting procedures for wound closure. During the period they remain open, special dressings are often used for wound care. Dressing material applied to an open wound serves to protect the wound from outside bacteria and other microbes, avoid dehydration of the wound surface, and encourage wound granulation. Many times, wet-to-dry dressings are placed; in this type of dressing, a gauze that has been moistened with normal saline or another solution is placed directly onto the wound surface or in the wound cavity, and a dry dressing is placed over this. The dressing is then loosely affixed to the skin using a nonirritating adhesive material.

Packing material such as iodoform or plain packing may also be used to fill a surgical wound cavity. By placing packing material into a cavity, the wound is able to granulate and heal progressively from the inside. Packing material aids in preventing the formation of a seroma or infection from developing. The wound packing is typically changed at least daily or more frequently until the cavity is small enough and packing is no longer necessary. Packing material comes in a variety of widths, including 1/4-inch, 1/2-inch, 1-inch, and 2-inch widths (Fig. 10.10).

Certain specialty dressings, such as vacuum-assisted closure (VAC) devices, require periodic changes of the dressing material. Whereas incisional wound VAC systems remain on the surgical wound for up to 7 days, standard wound VAC systems require regular care and change of the dressing materials, usually every 2 to 3 days. This usually requires removal of the on-site foam material, inspection of the wound for infection and proper wound granulation, and replacement of the foam material and dressing covering. A transition to wet-to-dry or a plain wound covering is usually made after there is sufficient granulation tissue noted in the wound.

SPECIAL CONSIDERATIONS: FOLEY CATHETER AND DRAIN MANAGEMENT

Foley catheters and surgical drains are often used and left in place at the end of a surgical procedure; however, they present an ongoing risk for infection when left indwelling over time. Catheter-associated urinary tract infection presents a significant risk to hospitalized patients and may be preventable by early and appropriate removal of Foley catheters after surgery.[17–19] Patients undergoing nonurological procedures should typically have their Foley catheters removed by postoperative day 1, with exception of patients presenting with an indwelling catheter or suprapubic tube prior to surgery, patients who are critically ill, and patients for whom accurate measurements of urine output is necessary.

Removal of surgical drains should also occur at the earliest feasible time to promote patient comfort and reduce the risk of SSI. Until then, periodic dressing changes should occur, inspecting the drain site at each dressing change for signs of infection. Prior to removal, drain fluid may be sent for creatinine, such as when a concern for urine extravasation exists; amylase and lipase when concern for a pancreatic injury exists; or triglycerides when concern for a chylous leak exists. For most small-caliber drains, a bandage placed over the drain site is sufficient, as the incision will close spontaneously. Larger drains may require skin closure, although this is usually unnecessary. One important consideration is for removal of a chest tube. To prevent a pneumothorax, the patient should inspire deeply as the chest tube is removed, and an airtight occlusive dressing should immediately be placed over the site.

REFERENCES

1. Gan TJ. Risk factors for postoperative nausea and vomiting. *Anesthesia and Analgesia.* 2006;102(6):1884–1898.
2. Sinclair DR, Chung F, Mezei G. Can postoperative nausea and vomiting be predicted? *Anesthesiology.* 1999;91(1): 109–118.
3. Carlisle JB, Stevenson CA. Drugs for preventing postoperative nausea and vomiting. *Cochrane Database of Systematic Reviews.* 2006;(3):CD004125.
4. Apfel CC, Korttila K, Abdalla M, et al. A factorial trial of six interventions for the prevention of postoperative nausea and vomiting. *New England Journal of Medicine.* 2004;350(24): 2441–2451.
5. Koretz RL, Avenell A, Lipman TO, Braunschweig CL, Milne AC. Does enteral nutrition affect clinical outcome? A systematic review of the randomized trials. *American Journal of Gastroenterology.* 2007;102(2):412–429. quiz 68.

6. Mariano E. Management of acute perioperative pain. In: Fanciullo G, ed. *UpToDate*. http://www.uptodate.com/contents/management-of-acute-perioperative-pain

7. Solomon D. NSAIDs: therapeutic use and variability of response in adults. In: Furst D, ed. *UpToDate*. http://www.uptodate.com/contents/nsaids-therapeutic-use-and-variability-of-response-in-adults

8. Rawlinson A, Kitchingham N, Hart C, McMahon G, Ong SL, Khanna A. Mechanisms of reducing postoperative pain, nausea and vomiting: a systematic review of current techniques. *Evidence-Based Medicine*. 2012;17(3):75–80.

9. Pontoppidan H. Mechanical aids to lung expansion in nonintubated surgical patients. *American Review of Respiratory Disease*. 1980;122(5 Pt 2):109–119.

10. Lawrence VA, Cornell JE, Smetana GW. Strategies to reduce postoperative pulmonary complications after noncardiothoracic surgery: systematic review for the American College of Physicians. *Annals of Internal Medicine*. 2006;144(8):596–608.

11. Liu Z, Tao X, Chen Y, Fan Z, Li Y. Bed rest versus early ambulation with standard anticoagulation in the management of deep vein thrombosis: a meta-analysis. *PloS One*. 2015;(4):10:e0121388.

12. Delaney CP, Zutshi M, Senagore AJ, Remzi FH, Hammel J, Fazio VW. Prospective, randomized, controlled trial between a pathway of controlled rehabilitation with early ambulation and diet and traditional postoperative care after laparotomy and intestinal resection. *Diseases of the Colon and Rectum*. 2003;46(7):851–859.

13. Oldmeadow LB, Edwards ER, Kimmel LA, Kipen E, Robertson VJ, Bailey MJ. No rest for the wounded: early ambulation after hip surgery accelerates recovery. *ANZ Journal of Surgery*. 2006;76(7):607–611.

14. Pua YH, Ong PH. Association of early ambulation with length of stay and costs in total knee arthroplasty: retrospective cohort study. *American Journal of Physical Medicine and Rehabilitation*. 2014;93(11):962–970.

15. Siu AL, Penrod JD, Boockvar KS, Koval K, Strauss E, Morrison RS. Early ambulation after hip fracture: effects on function and mortality. *Archives of Internal Medicine*. 2006;166(7):766–771.

16. Gould MK, Garcia DA, Wren SM, et al. Prevention of VTE in nonorthopedic surgical patients: Antithrombotic Therapy and Prevention of Thrombosis, 9th ed: American College of Chest Physicians Evidence-Based Clinical Practice Guidelines. *Chest*. 2012;141(2 suppl):e227S–e277S.

17. Fletcher KE, Tyszka JT, Harrod M, Fowler KE, Saint S, Krein SL. Qualitative validation of the CAUTI Guide to Patient Safety assessment tool. *American Journal of Infection Control*. 2016;44(10):1102–1109.

18. Parry MF, Grant B, Sestovic M. Successful reduction in catheter-associated urinary tract infections: focus on nurse-directed catheter removal. *American Journal of Infection Control*. 2013;41(12):1178–1181.

19. Pickard R, Lam T, MacLennan G, et al. Antimicrobial catheters for reduction of symptomatic urinary tract infection in adults requiring short-term catheterisation in hospital: a multicentre randomised controlled trial. *Lancet*. 2012;380(9857):1927–1935.

INDEX

Note: Page numbers followed by "f" indicate figures, "t" indicate tables, and "b" indicate boxes.